369 0213500

D1355617

Health Care Disparities
and the
LGBT Population

Health Care Disparities and the LGBT Population

Edited by Vickie L. Harvey
and Teresa Heinz Housel

LEXINGTON BOOKS
Lanham • Boulder • New York • Toronto • Plymouth, UK

www.rowman.com

10 Thornbury Road, Plymouth PL6 7PP, United Kingdom

British Library Cataloguing in Publication Information Available

Library of Congress Cataloging-in-Publication Data

Health care disparities and the LGBT population : health care disparities and the lgbt population / edited by Vickie L. Harvey and Teresa Heinz Housel.
    pages cm
  Includes bibliographical references and index.
   ISBN 978-0-7391-8702-9 (cloth : alk. paper) — ISBN 978-0-7391-8703-6 (electronic)
 1. Gays—Medical care—United States. 2. Bisexuals—Medical care—United States.
 3. Transgender people—Medical care—United States. 4. Health services accessibility—United States. 5. Discrimination in medical care—United States. I. Harvey, Vickie L., 1956- editor of compilation. II. Housel, Teresa Heinz, 1972- editor of compilation.
   RA564.9.H65H42 2014
   362.1086'64—dc23
   ISBN 978-1-4985-3605-9 (pbk : alk. paper)   2013049132

Contents

Part III: Silencing, Violence, and Other Forms of Intimidation of LGBT People

Foreword

Gary L. Kreps

For too long, lesbians, gay, bisexual, transgender, and questioning (LG-BTQ) people have been invisible and largely neglected populations of health care consumers, despite the fact that these different groups of people have many serious health concerns that need to be addressed. There has been almost no recognition within the health care system of the unique health issues and concerns that sexual minorities face on a daily basis. There is shockingly little sensitivity within the modern health care system to the serious problems with health care and health promotion efforts for sexual minority members. In fact, there are very few programs designed specifically to promote the health and to deliver high quality and culturally sensitive care to LGBTQ people.

Many LGBTQ individuals have avoided seeking health care services because of the history of rough, insensitive treatment they endure within health care delivery systems. Too often, sexual minorities are treated with disdain and suspicion by health care system workers. Worse, sexual minorities are often blamed for the health problems they face. There is often a tacit assumption made that their lifestyles and sexual orientations are primary causes for their ailments, regardless of whether there is any evidence for these assumptions. Many LGBTQ people are blamed for being sick, adding insult to injury! They are frequently treated with suspicion and fear, as potential carriers of infectious diseases. Due to neglect and prejudice, their health problems are often mis-diagnosed, and they consequently receive inappropriate treatments that only serve to exacerbate their ailments.

Reluctance to seek care from the health care system by LGBTQ people has resulted in late-term diagnoses for their health problems. This is a serious problem for many serious illnesses, such as cancers, HIV/AIDS, mental illnesses, and heart disease that are all best treated at early onset. For example, the later the stage of most cancers at time of diagnosis, the more difficult the cancers are to treat, especially if the disease has become metastatic (moved from an initial primary body site to secondary sites). Reluctance to seek care has also resulted in poor continuity of care for many sexual minorities. This is a serious problem because the best health care is a process of monitoring and refining treatments over time, especially for addressing long-term and chronic health problems. Reluctance to seek care, coupled with insensitively delivered health care services, can also reduce adherence with recommended treatments, therapies, and drug regimens for sexual minorities, dramatically reducing the effectiveness of these important treatments. Inevitably, reluctance to seek care leads to increased morbidity (sickness) and mortality (death) rates for LGBTQ people.

To improve health outcomes for LGBTQ people, the health care system needs to change, grow, learn, and become more culturally sensitive and supportive to the unique health needs and concerns of different groups of sexual minorities. First, it is important to note that sexual minority groups cannot be lumped together as though all group members have the same health issues and concerns. For example, lesbians have many very different health issues than those experienced by gay men. Transgender people also have particular health needs and concerns that need to be addressed. Even within these different sexual minority groups there are important health issue distinctions, based on age, ethnicity, and behavioral factors that need to be recognized and responded to. Health care providers and administrators need comprehensive and effective educational programs about the special health issues facing different sexual minorities and the best strategies for treating these health problems. Specialized health care protocols, programs, and treatment strategies need to be developed and implemented within modern health care systems to address the unique health care needs of sexual minorities.

Sensitivity and respect must be shown to all sexual minorities within the modern health care system! Many LGBTQ people may be understandably wary of the health care system. They may be worried about the social, political, and even criminal implications of full disclosure of their health issues to health care workers. They are likely to be suspicious about health care workers' motivations toward them. Care must be given to establishing trusting and supportive communication climates within health care systems, so sexual minorities feel cared for and as comfortable as possible. Genuine dialogue and active listening needs to be nurtured in the delivery of care. Kindness, sensitivity, and demonstration of cultural acceptance will go a long way to improving the delivery of care for sexual minorities.

Greater effort needs to be taken to promote the health for sexual minorities, who are heir to many unique health problems. It is always much better to prevent health problems than to treat those problems once they are experienced. Targeted and culturally sensitive health promotion campaigns need to be developed and implemented in collaboration with key members of sexual minority communities. Care must be taken to use appropriate language, examples, and motivational strategies in these campaigns to adequately meet the particular needs and communication orientations of carefully segmented groups of LGBTQ consumers. Efforts need to be taken to institutionalize health promotion programs within LGBTQ communities and to actively involve community members in the delivery of these programs to sustain health promotion efforts over time.

I am very excited about this new book that carefully examines the important health issues confronting LGBTQ populations. This is a book that has the potential to help raise consciousness and refine health practices. It is a book that is relevant reading for health care providers, health system administrators, health policy makers, health researchers, and health care consumers. Change is desperately needed within the modern health care system to enhance health outcomes for LGBTQ people, and I hope this book will help motivate needed improvements!

Gary L. Kreps, PhD
George Mason University

Foreword

Allan D. Peterkin

$\mathcal{A}$s I sat down to write this introduction for *Health Care Disparities and the LGBT Population,* I became keenly aware of a couple news items that caught my attention in the last few days. A young black trans woman was savagely beaten and killed in New York. The Russian Olympics were slated to go ahead despite the host country actively promoting a deeply offensive and deliberately provocative antigay message.

Then I remembered a well-intentioned colleague saying to me recently, "What's so different about gay and lesbian patients? I'm good with all my patients!" She's a fine doctor and may be right, but her comment still suggested a level of unfamiliarity with the facts, if not a benign form of heterosexism. In particular, most health care professionals still think that gender and sexual orientation are fixed, binary concepts and are ill prepared to deal candidly with sexuality in any of its expressions.

The field of population health reminds us that different groups of people have different health risks and vulnerabilities, their own unique definitions of risk, illness, health, and resilience, different perceptions (or fears of) health care, and differing levels of actual access to care. In addition, most of us don't subscribe to or even favor just one identity. Our queer identity can either collide with or enhance our spiritual, cultural, professional, social, and family lives.

If you ask most queer people across age groups and in most settings today, they can tell you that they have had at least one bad experience with clinics, hospitals, and health care providers. This can run from assumptions being made about who they were or "what they did sexually," to sloppy approaches to confidentiality, to being refused specific services or resources, to perceiving discomfort on the part of providers. Many can describe incidents where they encountered overtly expressed judgments of their sexuality or gender identity on "moral grounds." Patients with privilege (be it geographic in terms of the availability of other resources, financial, or related to a solid sense of selfhood and emotional resilience) find other caregivers and remain active, lifelong partners in their health care. Many others avoid going for routine checks, preventive care, educational updates, or counseling. The reasons for this are multiple and complex, but very often have to do with socioeconomic status, educational level, and cultural identity.

We can now identify specific demographic risks for queer men and women based on specific behaviors and strategize around things like safer sex, pap screening, and reducing smoking. However, the largest developmental risk for lesbians, gay, bisexual, and transgender (LGBT) individuals remains lifelong exposure to homophobic messaging, rejection, and physical violence because of their enduring effects on self-esteem, personal agency, and authenticity, and perceptions of self-worth. To this day, one of my goals as a psychotherapist, even in a Canadian health system providing universal access to care, is to convince certain people in my practice that they deserve to be treated with respect by those in their families, workplaces, cultural communities, places of worship, and health care teams. An equally important and more challenging message may be to convince them that loving themselves means taking good care of themselves in both body and mind.

Health Care Disparities effectively explores these complex inner and outer obstacles to access to care through the effective use of patient and client narratives, through canvassing the opinions of clinicians from multiple disciplines, and by including the voices of activists who have fought and still lobby for our right to comprehensive care with dignity for ourselves and our families. The formation of LGBT identity is explored along developmental lines from youth to adulthood to old age. Disparities in health care are named, and the real reasons for them (often disguised as "policy") are uncovered. We are asked to contemplate the many examples (intentional or unintended) where LGBT people do not feel accepted by those meant to care for them. This can start at the reception desk, continue with substandard intake forms, worsen in unwelcoming waiting rooms, and become unbearable due to a thoughtless question or remark from the nurse, doctor, or technician. Then there are the specialist referrals. Coming out to new providers is still an act of courage every single time and not without risk, as health care teams are only as strong as their weakest (or most arrogant, biased, or ignorant) link. A final and powerful section of the book examines the many situations in which LGBT individuals still feel silenced, threatened, or intimidated across the life span. This book fills a gap by providing engaging, authoritative, up-to-date information for health care trainees, practitioners, researchers, and policy makers, and is suitable for learners from all clinical disciplines at any level of training.

We all have a role to play in improving access to care. Reading *Health Care Disparities* is an important first step because it invites us to challenge our assumptions and identify gaps in knowledge. Even well-intentioned colleagues like the one I mentioned can do more to increase competence and attunement to the needs of LGBT people in their care.

Allan Peterkin, MD
University of Toronto

I

CONSTRUCTING IDENTITY
BY COMING OUT
TO YOUR PHYSICIAN

An Introduction to the Loosely Knit Patchwork of LGBT Health Care

Teresa Heinz Housel and Vickie L. Harvey

$\mathcal{A}$t the time of this writing, online health insurance marketplaces opened less than three weeks ago as part of Obama's Health Care Reform, colloquially referred to as ObamaCare, but officially called the Patient Protection and Affordable Care Act (PPACA). Each state has an exchange, which is a website intended to help people locate health coverage (Sun, 2013). This legislation that was signed into effect on March 23, 2010, is intended to reduce health care spending increases and provide affordable, quality care for all Americans (Klein, 2012). The Congressional Budget Office estimates that by 2022, PPACA would extend coverage to 33 million Americans by expanding the state-federal Medicaid program and giving low-income people government subsidies to buy coverage through insurance exchanges and marketplaces (Klein; NBC, 2010). The exchanges are intended to assist people who are uninsured, those who buy their own coverage, or people who decline their employer's insurance because is too costly or does not have certain needed benefits. The opening of the online marketplaces would allow millions of Americans to compare health plans online, find out if they are eligible to receive federal help with premiums, and purchase coverage.

These legislative reform efforts reflect the need for an overhaul of America's health care system. Although the richest nation in the world, the United States is one of only a few developed nations to lack a universal health care system for its residents (Fisher, 2012). According to Census Bureau data released in late 2010, more than 50 million Americans lack health insurance (NBC, 2010). This was the largest single-year increase since the census began tracking this statistic in 1987. Medicaid is intended to provide coverage for the nation's poor, but millions of Americans make too much to qualify for it and cannot afford private insurance premiums. Medicaid's strict guidelines also exclude many unemployed middle-class families who receive unemployment benefits. (NBC) Even for those who have a job, their employers might well not offer health care coverage as part of the employment package (Gould, 2012). A sizeable population of working but uninsured people includes those who are employed full-time and often have more than one job. Those jobs frequently include low-paid service positions without insurance or retirement benefits (Vieth & Jaworski, 2013). At the same time, the health care needs of America's rapidly increasing elderly population are sorely neglected. Many senior citizens cannot afford medication or are paying out of pocket due to the Medicaid part D prescription drug coverage gap (Kanavos & Gemmill-Toyama, 2010). These multiple examples of health care disparities are unconscionable in a country with such great wealth and world-renowned health providers and facilities.

In addition to the health care disparities described above, even Americans who are fortunate enough to have insurance do not have complete security in their coverage. For example, they could suddenly lose their coverage because insurance companies have no limits on raising premiums and companies can drop their clients for being sick or deny coverage for pre-existing conditions. Insurance companies can also stop treating people if they exceed their annual limit. These health care disparities reflect the need to improve a coverage system that is badly broken. The magnitude of changes proposed by the current health reform law is unparalleled and has the ability to change the lives of those who have been excluded from health insurance coverage. For the lesbian, gay, bisexual, and transgender, or LGBT, community in particular, these changes have the potential to radically increase access to coverage and care (Cray & Baker, 2013).

This co-edited volume of research addresses a population of people whose lack of health care access, mistreatment in health care settings, and refusal of health care services are often omitted from discussions about health care disparities and insurance reform. People who are LGBT are members of every community. They are diverse, come from all walks of life, and include people of all races and ethnicities, ages, socioeconomic statuses, and from all parts of the country. The perspectives and needs of LGBT people should be routinely considered in public health efforts to improve the overall health of every person and eliminate health disparities.

When we first developed the idea for this volume several years ago, we discussed the public debate around universal health care and the reasons why LGBT people are double-marginalized in the political and health care spheres. To consider just one example, we were greatly saddened to learn of the tragic case of Janice Langbehn and her partner of eighteen years, Lisa Pond (Parker-Pope, 2009, p. D5). Both were traveling with their children to Florida for a cruise vacation in February 2007 when Pond suddenly collapsed while taking photos of the kids playing basketball. During the frantic, harrowing events that followed, Pond was taken to a nearby hospital, where she was diagnosed with a brain aneurysm.

As Langbehn and the children waited in the trauma unit's waiting room, doctors provided almost no updates on Pond's condition until notifying Langbehn three hours later that there was no hope of recovery. Although Langbehn pleaded with hospital officials to visit her partner, she was only given a five-minute visit while a priest administered last rites. The children were not able to see their unconscious mother until midnight that day.

News of this tragic situation reached President Barack Obama, whose 2010 mandate led to the U.S. Department of Health and Human Services' new rules that nearly all U.S. hospitals offer visitation rights to same-sex partners (U.S. Department of Health & Human Services, 2010). By June 2013, the Human Rights Campaign, an advocacy group, reported that American hospitals were increasingly adopting policies banning discrimination against lesbian, gay, and bisexual patients and employees (Diep, 2013).

In the past decade, LGBT people have steadily made progress in securing equal civil rights in America. Fourteen states and Washington, D.C., now give same-sex couples at least some of the same rights afforded to heterosexual married couples (msn.com, 2013). Many heterosexual Americans are finally recognizing that LGBT people are a legitimate social minority that should have equal access to basic rights, opportunities, and responsibilities. National polling data indicate that the general public increasingly supports LGBT people having economic, political, and social equal rights (Pew Forum on Religion & Public Life, 2012). According to a Pew Forum on Religion & Public Life survey from November 2012, American public opinion slowly shifted toward supporting legalization of same-sex marriage. In 2001, Americans opposed same-sex marriage by a 57 percent to 35 percent margin. In 2012, 48 percent supported same-sex marriage, while 43 percent of polled Americans opposed it. This same Pew study from 2012 study reported that Millennials (people born in 1981 or later) are almost twice as likely (64 percent) to support same-sex marriage as the Silent Generation (those born between 1928–1945) at 33 percent.

This opinion shift mirrors the policy changes at the state and national levels. Thirteen American states and Washington, D.C., currently have legal same-sex marriage. Seven states now currently allow civil unions and domestic partnerships, which are similar to marriage in that they confer legal status and rights at the state level. However, civil unions and domestic partnerships may not be recognized by other states or the federal government (msn.com, 2013). Twenty-five states do not allow gay marriages or civil unions of any sort according state law and/or gay marriage is banned by state constitution.

For the remaining states, it's more complicated (msn.com). For example, Wisconsin allows gay couples to register as domestic partners, allowing some legal benefits such as hospital visitation rights. However, their domestic partnership law is one of the most limited in the country. Gay marriage has been banned by constitutional amendment in Wisconsin since 2006. LGBT advocates have been pushing for gay marriage especially hard after their neighboring state of Minnesota approved gay marriage. Unfortunately, experts say the state is not likely to revisit the issue anytime soon (msn.com). This legalization of rights also places these states along a similar trajectory as other countries such as the South Africa, Canada, and Sweden, which allow same-sex couples to marry. Additional countries such as Austria and New Zealand allow civil unions rights that under law are identical to marriage, but same-sex couples cannot legally adopt in those countries.

In the United States, more than twenty-one states now offer nondiscrimination protections based on sexual orientation, gender identity, or both in regard to employment (Human Rights Campaign, 2012). These rates improve in health care situations. In almost half of American states, discriminating against LGBT patients is illegal. Twenty-two states have laws that prohibit discrimination based on a person's sexual orientation in "public accommodations," meaning most businesses that serve the public. Public accommodations include the provision of health care services by physicians, hospitals, and other health care providers. Fourteen of these twenty-two states also prohibit public accommodations discrimination based on a person's gender identity (Clifford, Hertz, & Doskow, 2012).

The divergent opinions on civil rights for LGBT people in American society mirrors how their everyday experiences are marked by discrimination, particularly in the health sector. Previous research suggests that LGBT people experience worse health outcomes than their heterosexual counterparts (Krehely, 2009). Differences in sexual behavior account for some of these disparities, but others are associated with social and structural inequities, such as the stigma and discrimination that LGBT populations experience (U.S. Department of Health & Human Services, 2012). The health outcomes result from factors such as low rates of health insurance coverage, high rates of stress due to systematic harassment, stigma, and discrimination, and a lack of cultural competency in the health care system (Krehely). In particular, LGBT individuals in general report experiencing stigma because of wider social devaluation of same-sex relationships (Frost, 2011). As a result, this stigma, stress, and trauma frequently manifest in negative health-related behaviors such as smoking and excessive drinking, and in health conditions such as obesity, depression, and health disease (Lewis, Derlega, Griffin, & Krowinski, 2003). The National Coalition for LGBT Health reports that health disparities are highest for LGBT people who are also racial or ethnic minorities because of their double minority status. Transgender individuals, and especially minority transgender people, tend to be uninsured, or even if they have coverage, cannot obtain services because most policies contain transgender-specific exclusions (Cray & Baker, 2012). Due to the lack of consistent data collection on sexual identity, we can only estimate the extent of LGBT health disparities (Krehely).

As we developed this volume's concept, we realized that more empirical research is badly needed to examine LGBT people's experiences in the health-care context. This lack of data collection on sexual orientation and identity in state and federal health care surveys has led to inadequate information about LGBT populations. This paucity of data hinders researchers' ability to best understand LGBT people's health needs and also impedes the establishment of health programs and public policies that benefit them.

Given this background of discrimination, this volume's research will increase people's understanding of the social and structural discrimination that LGBT populations experience. The essays' diverse perspectives will benefit health care professionals, faculty, staff, and activists working at diverse types of institutions with LGBT people. In addition, some authors are members of the LGBT community and/or have firsthand experience with health care disparities. Sexual orientation and gender identity experiences profoundly shape a person's social and structural transition into health care and heavily determine what barriers to health care and health coverage he or she will face.

Taken together, this volume's three sections address important issues in this evolving research area. The first section, "Constructing Identity by Coming Out to Your Physician," examines the complex doctor-patient relationship dynamics when patients reveal their sexual orientation to physicians. As this section's essays illustrate, LGBT people too often experience hurtful comments and are refused treatment by physicians when they disclose their sexual orientation. There is much cultural competency improvement to be done as physicians learn how to sensitively and professionally approach sexual orientation.

The second section, "Access, Disparities, and Harassment Under the Guise of Policies," considers the important issue of health care coverage. Same-sex couples, and especially those who make less income or are trans-sexual, tend to lack insurance coverage. Insurance reform must address this coverage gap because LGBT people are more likely to experience stressors that lead to health problems. This correlation is heightened by the fact that physicians sometimes do not treat LGBT patients, or if they do, give them substandard treatment.

The health care disparities are further affirmed through verbal and other communicative acts that silence LGBT people. To this end, the last section,

"Silencing, Violence, and Other Forms of Intimation of LGBT People," examines the multiple ways in which LGBT people are intimidated. Although silencing has the usual goal of closing off the target's opportunities for self-actualization, silencing can also generate activism.

This book will ultimately benefit not only LGBT people but will also more broadly improve the lives of entire communities, medical care, and prevention programs and services. Discrimination in health care is unacceptable. This volume's essays collectively make the case for improved government investment in training programs around LGBT health issues, reducing LGBT health disparities, and helping providers become culturally competent by providing insider perspectives on LGBT health disparities. Improvements to our country's health care system should go beyond providing universal insurance and should ensure equitable health care for all.

The Importance of Sexual Orientation Disclosure to Physicians for Women Who Have Sex with Women

Karina Willes and Mike Allen

$\mathcal{T}$he doctor/patient interaction lies at the heart of the practice of medicine. The doctor obtains information from a patient to identify symptoms, understand history, and provide recommendations for diagnosis and treatment. Conversely, the patient needs to believe that disclosures made by the patient do not adversely impact the quality of care or negatively affect elements of the relationship. This chapter considers how women who have sex with women (WSW) obtain medical care and select physicians. The decision to disclose sexual practices to a medical professional by a woman carries a number of implications for the provision of health care.[1]

The concept of human sexuality is made up of three components: attraction, behavior, and identity (O'Hanlan, Dibble, Hagan, & Davids, 2004, p. 227). WSW focuses on the behavioral aspects of sexuality for women who have sex with other women. The term WSW includes women who may identify themselves as lesbian, heterosexual, gay, straight, bisexual, queer, or may prefer not to identify with any sexual identity. The term describes a behavior that a woman engages in with another woman without addressing the issues of identity.

WSW look like everyone else (no specific race, age, socioeconomic background, or geographical location), act like anyone else, and possess no identifiable or unique characteristic. This adds to the complexity of identifying WSW patients and the need for physicians to thoughtfully inquire into a patient's sexual orientation or behavior (Rankow, 1995, p. 486; Stevens, Tatum, & White, 1996, p. 122).

In twenty-two U.S. states, laws specifically prohibit doctors, hospitals, and medical facilities from refusing to treat a person due to sexual orientation. Therefore, in twenty-eight states the law does not prohibit refusal to treat LGBT patients (NOLO Law for All, 2013). Likewise, hospitals or clinics may be supported or affiliated with religious organizations that do not support LGBT relationships. The religious affiliations create a fear of discrimination. The American Medical Association (AMA) policy promotes education for medical students about LGBT issues, but this type of training is not a requirement (Moyer, 2011). What this means for WSW is that access to care without the fear of discrimination may not exist in some places and has unclear status in others. For this reason, many WSW may not identify sexual practices to the primary caregiver for fear of a negative reaction. Such fears may be rooted in previous experience with the medical community by purposeful, thoughtless, or inadvertent actions.

Nondisclosure of sexual practices may not play an important role when treating an upper respiratory infection or conditions not directly related to one's sexual identity. One would be hard-pressed to argue that a person's sexuality would play a direct role in whether or not the person requires any change in diagnosis or treatment for a cold. However, other illnesses and conditions may have a higher or lower risk related to the person's sexuality. Additionally, discussions about reproduction and the inclusion or identification of the significant other (spouse) may differ based on the woman's sexual orientation. This chapter considers how the failure of identification to a health care professional may impact the quality health care practices as well as the feelings of the woman seeking care. The attitudes and predispositions of both the patients and the health care providers in this situation play a role that impacts the standard of care provided/received.

The hetero-normative assumptions that society has about relationships permeate the medical setting where patient information forms and verbal questions reflect assumptions about sexuality that are inaccurate or incomplete. When a WSW patient is asked questions such as whether or not she is sexually active and about the type of contraception used, the responses may contain important missing or misleading information (Rankow, 1995, p. 488). A lesbian could be very sexually active with multiple partners with no need for contraceptive advice, despite the answers provided on many standard patient questionnaires about sexuality.

HISTORICAL PERSPECTIVE OF WSW PATIENT SEXUAL ORIENTATION AND THE PRACTICE OF MEDICINE

In the late 1980s, the World Health Organization (WHO) was convinced to remove homosexuality from the International Classification of Diseases (Adams, 1989). As Adams states, "Given this history, it's not surprising that the current relationship between lesbians and medicine is an uncomfortable one" (p. 53).

Within the last three decades, disclosure of sexual orientation to medical providers frequently generated the risk of negative consequences. Just three decades ago, during the 1980s, several studies found that health care providers felt uncomfortable treating gay patients, pathologized homosexuality, and felt that homosexuality was immoral (Adams, 1989; Stevens, 1994). Taking a look at a few studies from the 1980s and 1990s provides valuable perspective on patients' disclosure of sexual orientation.

An early groundbreaking study by Johnson, Guenther, Laube, and Keettel (1981) conducted in the United States on lesbian and bisexual women found that 40 percent of the participants believed that disclosing sexual orientation would adversely affect the quality of their general health care. Only 18 percent of the participants disclosed sexual orientation to a physician, while 49 percent said that they would like to do so. Additionally, 77 percent of the respondents indicated that they would like to discuss sexual problems with a physician if they found one who was comfortable with lesbian patients. The vast majority (94 percent) of the respondents indicated that they would prefer a lesbian physician. Finally, 63 percent of the respondents stated a physician visit would be more comfortable if a friend or advocate could come with them.

Smith, Johnson, and Guenther (1985) specifically studied gynecological care attitudes and experiences for WSW. The study analyzed the results of a questionnaire distributed at cultural events for women residing in the United States and Canada in 1980. Forty percent of respondents believed physician knowledge of sexual orientation would negatively impact health care. Likewise, 30 percent of the respondents, although wanting to, did not disclose orientation to their physicians (Smith, Johnson, & Guenther, p. 1087).

Later in the 1980s, Cochran and Mays (1988) conducted a study focusing on black lesbian and bisexual women. This study found that only 33 percent of lesbians spoke openly with physicians about sexual orientation. Bisexual women were even less likely to discuss the topic. Many participants reported that although sexual orientation was never discussed, the patients believed that the physician knew about their sexual orientation. If this is taken into account, 44 percent of lesbians and 27 percent of bisexuals believed the physician knew the participant's sexual orientation (Cochran & Mays, p. 618).

From the physician's perspective, a survey of 700 members of the American Association of Physicians for Human Rights in 1994, just a few years after the WHO declassified homosexuality, found that 66 percent of the respondents observed colleagues providing substandard or denying care to lesbian, gay, or bisexual patients, and 50 percent of respondents observed situations where care was denied to homosexual patients (McCormick,

1994; Rankow, 1995, p. 486). Likewise, 88 percent reported that they heard colleagues using disparaging language when speaking about LGB patients (Rankow, p. 486).

Reasons for Nondisclosure of Sexual Orientation

In Polek and Hardie's (2010) recent study focusing on lesbians' knowledge of human papillomavirus (HPV) risk, they found that only 52 percent of the study's participants, bisexual, or transgender women in Delaware disclosed sexual orientation to health care providers. Another 6 percent disclosed only after the health care provider asked. This study goes on to show that there was a far greater likelihood of a lesbian patient who disclosed sexual orientation to her health care provider of not knowing the risk of woman-to-woman transmission of HPV. Although the study does not provide an explanation of this, it proposes that this may be a symptom of biased care as a result of the sexual orientation disclosure. The question people must ask themselves when meeting and seeking health advice from physicians is how the physician providing care may react to disclosure of any personal information. Previous experience with the health care system or the stories told by friends often provide the basis for the expectations about why WSW patients believe that the physician reacts poorly.

Anyone seeking health care must consider the possible implications of self-disclosure on that care. A survey sponsored by the National Lesbian Health Organization and conducted by Harris Interactive and the Mautner Project (2005) found that 16 percent of lesbians delayed seeking health care because they feared discrimination based on sexual orientation. Likewise, 74 percent of lesbians who experienced discrimination in a physician's office believed the discrimination resulted from sexual orientation (DeBold, 2007, p. 2).

The acceptance of a partner participating or being a part of any health care decision or practice plays a significant role for many WSW. The need to identify a patient as part of a same-sex couple or a patient's partner as the contact person or the person from whom social support is provided may cause difficulties in the health care setting. In many states a lesbian couple cannot legally marry or have a civil union. The status of any partner in a permanent relationship becomes unclear and difficult in some cases to understand. De-Bold (2007) states, "Informed and open discussions regarding all aspects of a patient's life (including relationship status) promote health, prevent disease, and improve access to and the quality of health care" (p. 7). The need to discuss reproductive or end-of-life issues takes on significance when the partner is of the same gender. Decisions about medical care and the provision of social support during an illness or recovery from a stroke, heart attack, or accident become something necessary to consider as a couple and the partner of the patient should be included. If the couple was a married heterosexual couple, the expectation of inclusion of the partner would be virtually assured as well as the family and in-laws. For a lesbian couple that is not permitted to marry, the status of these issues becomes clouded and uncertain. At a minimum, the lesbian couple would need to create legal documentation such as designating a health care power of attorney and writing a living will to ensure that as many rights are maintained as possible during medical emergencies. Some couples will keep these documents on-hand, in glove boxes, or filed with primary care physicians (PCP) to avoid a situation where one partner would not be allowed to visit or make medical decisions should her partner require support or assistance. One critical question to consider is how the medical care provider handles these issues. Even in states where same sex couples can marry, the reaction of medical professionals and institutions may not be universally supportive.

As of August 2013, approximately 43 percent of the U.S. population lives in states allowing same-sex marriage or some form of civil union or domestic partnership rights (Freedom to Marry, 2013), as shown in table 2.1:

Table 2.1.

States Allowing Same-Sex Marriage	States Allowing Civil Union or Domestic Partnership
• California	• Colorado (Civil Union)
• Connecticut	• Hawaii (Civil Union)
• Delaware	• Illinois (Civil Union)
• Iowa	• New Jersey (Civil Union)
• Maine	• Oregon (Domestic Partnership)
• Maryland	• Nevada (Domestic Partnership)
• Massachusetts	• Wisconsin (Limited Domestic Partnership)
• Minnesota	
• New Hampshire	
• New York	
• Rhode Island	
• Vermont	
• Washington	
• Washington, DC	

Clinical Implications of Nondisclosure of Sexual Orientation

Before understanding the clinical implications of nondisclosure of sexual orientation, a physician needs to understand the complexity of sexual orientation for WSW. Numerous studies over the three decades indicate that although a WSW may identify as lesbian, she may have engaged in heterosexual sexual activities in the past or, in some cases, recently. In many cases, heterosexual sexual activities occur for WSW younger in life, while the woman is struggling with sexual identity issues. In fact, 75 to 90 percent of WSW studied reported sexual activity with men (Rankow, 1995; Bradford, Ryan, & Rothblum, 1994; Cochran & Mays, 1988; Johnson et al., 1981). Because the assumed sexual identity of WSW, particularly those who identify as lesbian, infers no heterosexual activity, a medical provider may incorrectly assume that a patient has sex only with women. Knowledge of a patient's sexual orientation or practices often impacts the appropriate diagnosis, counseling, and care of patients with medical concerns.

Focusing on specific medical conditions, research demonstrates different risk factors affecting patient health that impact WSW. Some evidence exists that lesbians are more likely to become impacted by some medical conditions. To this end, certain risk factors are often widespread among lesbians. Obesity is more common among lesbian women than heterosexual women (DeBold, 2007, p. 3; Boehmer, Bowen, & Bauer, 2007, p. 1137; Boehmer & Bowen, 2009, p. 360). There are also higher rates of alcohol consumption and smoking for lesbians as compared to heterosexual women (Bradford et al., 1994, p. 239; O'Hanlan et al., 2004, p. 228). These factors weigh into higher incidents of cardiovascular disease and certain types of cancer, including cervical, ovarian, and breast cancer (White & Dull, 1997).

Lesbians use oral contraceptives less frequently than heterosexual women and are more frequently nulliparous, having never been pregnant or given birth to a baby. These conditions correlate to increased incidents of gynecological cancers (e.g., ovarian, endometrial, cervical, and breast) (Dibble, Roberts, Robertson, & Paul, 2002, p. E1; O'Hanlan et al., 2004, p. 228). The study conducted by Dibble et al. found that lesbians also had higher BMIs, which contributes to the development of many cancers.

The Institute of Medicine (IOM) released a report in 1999 entitled, "Lesbian Health: Current Assessment and Directions for the Future." This report concludes that, at the time, there weren't any specific health conditions that were more or less prevalent to the lesbian community. It simply stated that lesbian women experienced the same health conditions that all women experience (Solarz, 1999, p. 6). However, more recent studies have begun to reexamine this premise, focusing on specific health conditions affecting women, and thus they contradict the earlier assertion. Although WSW experience the same health conditions that all women face, risk factors and sexual practices may lead to higher or lower likelihood of developing some conditions (Smith et al., 1985, p. 1085). For example, Marrazzo and Gorgos (2012) found in the United States, bacterial vaginosis (a common bacterial infection of the vagina) was prevalent in 45 percent of WSW, while only prevalent in 29 percent of heterosexual women (p. 207).

Furthermore, misconceptions exist about the risk of sexually transmitted infections (STIs) for lesbian women. Many WSW believe that they are at a lower risk of contracting an STI. However, bacterial or viral infections, such as bacterial vaginosis, HIV, and herpes can all be passed through sexual practices common during lesbian sex (e.g., sharing insertive sex toys, digital-genital, digital-anal, oral-genital, oral-anal, and genital-genital contact-tribadism) (Marrazzo, Coffey, & Bingham, p. 2005).

Polek and Hardie (2010) found that 30 percent of lesbians surveyed either did not know or did not believe that HPV could be transmitted between women (p. E191). Similarly, an early study, Johnson et al. (1981) indicated that cervical dysplasia was much lower among WSW, and generally only affected WSW identifying as bisexual. This same study found that monilial vaginitis (yeast infection) occurred at lower rates than for heterosexual women, and questioned the validity of responses from three women who reported contracting trichomoniasis (a common STD) while only sexual active with other women (Johnson et al., p. 23). Because of the belief that WSW are lower risk for these types of conditions than heterosexual women, WSW use few precautions to avoid infection. WSW fail to routinely use barriers such as dental dams, gloves, or condoms. They may also fail to focus on hygienic precautions such as washing hands or washing shared sex toys (Marrazzo et al., 2005, p. 6).

The result of sexual orientation disclosure and understanding a patient's sexual history and sexual behavior helps physicians consider appropriate diagnoses and eliminate those that may be inappropriate (Cochran & Mays, 1988, p. 616). Knowledge of a patient's sexual orientation impacts the types of questions relevant to that patient's health history. In order to establish rapport and trust with a patient, a physician needs to ask questions related to the patient's life experience. Stevens, Tatum, and White (1996) provide suggestions for providing optimal care for lesbian patients. The authors encourage health care providers to dispel myths STD transmission, eliminate bias and heterosexist assumptions in questions asked of patients, and "take disclosure in stride" (Stevens et al., p. 127). Likewise, the lack of knowledge of the patient's sexual orientation does not permit the customization of treatment and creates less effective medical care. The fear of discrimination or reduced quality of care makes the WSW patient less likely to disclose sexual orientation to any health care provider.

Selection of a Health Care Provider

Like any other person, WSW want a health care provider who will provide high quality care. When concerns about any part of a person's identity play a role in health care, the selection of a doctor becomes a central focus. One question is how WSW select or identify an LGBT-friendly doctor; in other words, one who openly accepts LGBT patients. The obvious solution is to ask WSW friends about the places and persons that provide care without the fear of discrimination or rejection based on a self-disclosure.

Mulligan and Heath (2007) studied bisexual, queer, and lesbian–identified women in Australia. The participants of this study were more likely to carefully seek health care providers who were more accepting. In fact, the participants listed this acceptance of sexuality to be the primary consideration when selecting a health care provider. The participants considered open-mindedness and being "friendly toward people of different sexual orientations" to be a feature of good service (Mulligan & Heath, p. 470).

WSW are more likely to disclose their sexual orientation to health care providers who do not discriminate against lesbians or exhibit lesbian sensitivity. Lesbians will often look for clues in the provider's office as to whether they are in a "safe" health care environment, or if the health care provider may harm them, should they decide to disclose (St. Pierre, 2012, p. 201). Word-of-mouth referrals, or the snowball technique, also represent a way for a community to provide information to members about the quality of services provided. Essentially, one woman can answer questions from other women about where to go to receive quality care. Likewise, LGBT community centers may provide directories of health care or other professional service providers who are either LGBT or allies. White and Levinson (1995) first considered the issues of how to create a medical history interview environment in which WSWs feel comfortable and are willing to discuss their sexual practices and history.

Many health care organizations now provide for web, text, or video information from doctors and other providers about each provider's approach and philosophy to health care. The question about whether and how a physician can identify themselves as LGBT-friendly remains an element of decision making. Obviously a doctor identifying themselves as open to persons of diverse sexuality can provide more confidence in the decision about the choice of a provider.

What follows is a survey of WSWs that provides a basis for understanding how they go about selecting a doctor. The issue of discrimination, of whether to disclose, and how to determine what they believe the reaction of the caregiver, all play a central role in shaping the orientation and reaction to care.

METHODS

WSWs were recruited for this study through the use of Facebook, Twitter, and email to complete an electronic survey in May, June, and part of July 2013. Likewise, Facebook postings were made on several lesbian-centric or LGBT social group walls, and emails were sent to various LGBT center contacts. Additional participants were recruited in person at Pridefest, in Milwaukee, Wisconsin, on June 7–9, 2013, by passing out flyers containing a link to the survey to potential WSW.

The survey contained three types of questions: demographic, medical care experience, and physician selection. The questions used an equal mix of both open-ended, text-based questions, and yes-no questions to attempt to capture participant stories and impressions that would explain the quantitative data provided. To be included in the data analysis, the person had to indicate that she has biological gender that is not male and that she has sex with women.

Participants were asked to identify a sexual orientation: heterosexual, homosexual, bisexual, asexual, queer, other. The medical experience questions delved into a participant's experiences with a PCP and an obstetrician/gynecologist (OB/GYN). The final group of questions asked participants to identify the preferred method for selecting physicians, whether or not online tools are used in the process, and whether or not a physician's acceptance of LGBT patients, or identity of being LGBT or an ally, is considered during selection.

Of the 220 respondents, 82 percent (178) indicated they have sex with women only, while 18 percent (39) indicated that they have sex with both men and women. When asked to identify sexual orientation, 73 percent (158) identified as homosexual (including the terms lesbian and gay), 13 percent (28) identified as bisexual, 12 percent (25) reported as queer, one indicated she refused to label her sexual orientation, and one identified as asexual.

Age was reported by 206 participants with a range from 18 to 64: 13 percent (18–24), 30 percent (25–34), 31 percent (35–44), 21 percent (45–54), and 6 percent (55–64). Thirty-four percent of respondents reported earning less than $40,000, 44 percent reported earning between $40,000 and $100,000, and 22 percent reported incomes from $100,000 and higher. Seventy-one percent (152) reported being employed full-time, while the remaining reported part-time employment, retired, unemployed, or full-time student statuses.

In some demographic respects, the pool of respondents was somewhat homogenous. Approximately 78 percent indicated their ethnic background to be Caucasian or white, including those who indicated European, German, English, American, and various other groupings of European descent. Nine percent of respondents indicated their ethnic background to be African American, Black, or African descent. The remaining group of respondents indicated Hispanic/Latina (including Cuban or Puerto Rican), multi- or biracial backgrounds, or Asian, Jewish, or Pacific Islander. The majority, 85 percent, indicated they lived in either a metropolitan or suburban area, while 15 percent reported living in a rural area. Seventy-one percent of the respondents reported being employed full-time. Sixty-five percent of the respondents indicated that they were in committed relationship, including being engaged, married, or in a domestic partnership. Seventy percent reported earning an associate degree or higher. Sixty percent reported having a bachelor's degree or higher. Twenty-eight percent reported master's degrees or higher. Eightynine percent (178) of the respondents reported having insurance, while 11 percent (23) did not. Slightly less than half of the participants reported their current state as being Wisconsin, with all others coming from 29 other states, Canada, and Europe. Although a significant portion of participants are from Wisconsin, when comparing the results between the sample from Wisconsin and the sample from all of the other states and countries, no significant difference in responses were noted.

RESULTS

Participants' Routine Health Care

The health care experience portion of the survey began by questioning where the participants normally seek health care. Eighty-four percent (106) indicated they seek care from a PCP's office, while the remaining 15 percent (33) responded with walk-in clinic, emergency room, or other (including places such as Walgreen's walk-in or free clinics).

When asked if the participant had a PCP, 82 percent (171) responded that they did, while 18 percent (37) responded that they did not. More than half of the respondents, 57 percent (97) indicated that they have had a relationship with the PCP for three or more years. Of the 37 without a current PCP, 86 percent (32) indicated that although they currently do not have a PCP, they had a PCP in the past. Only 2 percent (5) have never had a PCP. Those that do not have a PCP were asked why they did not and most responded with items such as "no insurance," "can't afford," or responses that indicated either the participant has recently moved and hasn't yet found a new doctor or the doctor has retired or moved recently and has not yet been replaced.

When asked if the participant had an OB/GYN, 53 percent (107) indicated that they did, while 47 percent (94) indicated that they did not. Forty-eight percent of the respondents with an OB/GYN indicated they have had a relationship with that physician for three or more years. Of those 94 respondents without an OB/GYN, 49 percent (46) indicated that they have had an OB/GYN in the past, while the remaining 51 percent (48) have not. The majority of those who did not currently have an OB/GYN provided reasons such as "no insurance" or "I use my primary doctor for everything" for not using that specialty medical provider.

Are WSW Disclosing to Physicians?

The survey asked whether or not PCPs or OB/GYNs knew about the respondent's sexual orientation. Regarding disclosure to PCPs, 73 percent (147) of respondents indicated that the physician did know the participant's orientation. The remaining 27 percent (55) responded that their PCP did not know the participant's orientation. Although many of the responses indicated rather general, nonspecific reasons for the lack of disclosure, some examples provide interesting insight into the perception of physician bias. One respondent wrote, "The physician encouraged me to stay celibate until I found 'the man I will marry.' I did not feel safe disclosing any of my sexual history, let alone my sexual orientation." Another respondent stated, "I think she will judge me and all she talked about was her husband and church . . . I'm not going to her in the future." Many of the reasons provided indicated that the topic has never come up or that it wasn't an issue that was relevant to the care being provided by the PCP.

A relatively common response for the PCP not knowing the sexual orientation, one that seems innocuous at first, was simply that it "didn't come up" in conversation. This type of response could reflect the general hesitance to ask on the physician's side as well as the hesitancy to reveal on the patient's side. One may ask is the reason that the topic of sexual orientation was not approached in conversations because the patient feared to disclose or that the physician was too uncomfortable to ask?

The level of disclosure was slightly higher for participants with their OB/GYNs, with 82 percent (123) indicating that the physician did know their orientation while 18 percent (28) did not. The participants were asked to provide a reason for the lack of disclosure. Several responses provided meaningful context to the issues being examined. One participant wrote, "I don't think it is a factor in my health. I don't feel that I need to disclose it as I've had a previous experience where the OB/GYN was told and it was very uncomfortable." Another indicated, "I was married to a man at the time and was still in the 'closet.'" A third respondent simply stated, "I was afraid to tell."

The survey inquired as to whether or not the participant "ever feared or hesitated" disclosing her sexual orientation to any physician. Fifty-two percent (106) of the participants indicated that they have, while 48 percent (97) said that they have not. Twenty-nine (30 percent) responses specifically mentioned a fear of a physician's judgment. One response plainly states, "Gays aren't exactly accepted everywhere. Sometimes, they are not so nice." Twenty-one (22 percent) respondents feared that a doctor knowing would adversely affect the quality of care or treatment received. A participant stated, "I feared them not understanding and/or making judgments that might impact my quality of care." Another wrote, "I felt I would not get the same care as someone who was straight." Fourteen (14 percent) of the women felt a general discomfort about disclosure. Others indicated that they feared the doctor's reaction, were fearful due to past experiences, hesitated due to the doctor already making assumptions, feared not being accepted, or feared it would become part of their record. One respondent stated that she "didn't want it in my record didn't feel comfortable with the physician." Another insightful response indicated, "Awkwardness. She assumed so easily that I had a boyfriend it was weird to interrupt and correct her."

Another respondent explained her reluctance to disclose including her past personal experience:

> After I told my last doctor that I was gay, she came back in and it was the quickest, most rushed pap smear I have had, and hurt. I felt like she was rushing, though there was no one in the waiting room. I felt uncomfortable. I have also had to pay for a pregnancy test that I told them I did not need, even after I told them I was gay. I did not realize that was what they were doing until I got the bill and saw that I had to pay for a pregnancy test, "because it is procedure." So now I often don't feel comfortable, especially when a doctor may start by asking if I have a boyfriend. I find myself shutting down right then.

The participants were asked through several different questions if they have experienced bias, through a doctor becoming uncomfortable after disclosure, through experiencing general bias (not specified), or if they feel they have ever received a lower quality of care because of sexual orientation. Twenty-seven percent (52) responded that they have experienced a physician becoming uncomfortable after learning their sexual orientation. Examples noting the perception of a doctor becoming uncomfortable include:

> "I went to student health services to get tested for mono because my girlfriend was diagnosed with it and I had not been feeling well. When she asked why I thought I had it, I explained that I might have gotten it

from my girlfriend. She didn't understand at first, but then looked at me disgusted when she did understand."

"It was an ER visit and the 'doors slammed' in his eyes when he realized my 'friend' was actually my spouse. The visit became very impersonal after that."

"The doctor traded his visit with another doctor as he was uncomfortable about it."

"I disclosed my sexual orientation (including my partner's trans status to my old family physician who I had growing up in a small town), in order to clarify that birth control was not necessary at the present time. He reacted with genuine surprise and confusion, and then asked me whether my father knew about this and what he would think if he knew."

Seventeen percent (33) indicated that they believed they had experienced bias. Eleven percent (21) indicated they perceived that they have received a lower quality of care due to their sexual orientation. One participant offered her experience that a doctor was "not willing to help me with infertility issues because the doctor was biased about lesbians raising children."

Finally, participants were asked if they have ever felt the need to exclude partners from health care experiences. Fourteen percent (27) felt the need to exclude a partner. One response introduced a religious aspect to a health care experience, "I was admitted to a Catholic hospital and even though we have advance directives, the doctor was clearly religious and we were not comfortable having her [the respondent's partner] 'complicate' things."

How Is Sexual Orientation Disclosed?

When asked how the participant disclosed her sexual orientation to her PCP, 30 percent (41) participants indicated that they disclosed their orientation to the physician during a conversation about sexual activity. More than half of those participants, 17 percent (24), indicated they disclosed verbally during a conversation about birth control or in response to pregnancy test requests. Twenty-four percent (34) either disclosed that they had female partners, brought their partners with them to the appointment, or indicated either the doctor knew their partners or they brought their partners with them to the visit. The remaining participants indicated that they disclosed their sexual orientation on the form provided by the physician's office, while discussing family planning, or through general, nondescript conversation or that she did not remember.

The results were similar for how the participant disclosed her sexual orientation to an OB/GYN. Twenty-six percent (30) participants indicated that they disclosed during a conversation with their physician regarding sexual activity. Eleven of those responses were specifically related to conversations about birth control. Seven percent (9) participants stated that they either disclosed that they had a female partner or the physician already knew their female partner. Four participants disclosed during a conversation about starting a family or for obstetric care. The remaining participants stated they told their doctor while discussing family-planning or obstetric care, or during general conversation. Several participants indicated that their OB/GYN was the same physician as their PCP.

Why Do WSW Believe Physicians Should Know?

The participants were asked if they felt it was important for a physician to know their sexual orientation. Eighty-four percent (167) indicated that they believed knowing the sexual orientation was important.

Some examples of why the participants felt it is important for a physician to be aware of her sexual orientation include:

"To treat me as a whole person, they would need to know the whole story."

"They need to know as much as possible about you to provide the best care to you, this is just one more piece of information that helps them."

"Certain illnesses are more or less prevalent depending on your orientation."

"So that the doctor does not say things that are not relevant like 'what kind of birth control do you use' or 'do you have painful intercourse.'"

"It is also sometimes nice for that information to be out in the open so that I don't have to feel subjected to my doctor's hetero-normative assumptions."

"You can't have secrets from the doctor. If you have a health care proxy and it states your partner as your proxy it also states your relationship to that proxy. I wouldn't want something to happen and the doctor tell my wife 'I need to speak to her relatives now.'"

One participant expressed frustration with the assumptions often made with WSW patients, "Maybe I am tired of being asked if I use birth control though now I am finally too old and people have stopped asking! I don't know. My partner is also my power of health care attorney. I also think people need to be educated and avoid making assumptions."

How Do WSW Search for Physicians?

The survey specifically questioned the process of searching for physicians through online or Web-based methods. Participants were asked to describe the process used to find a new physician. Responses such as, "ask family and friends," "ask people I know and trust," "I'm asking my friends who are lesbians," or "word of mouth," were common.

Participants indicated that conducting online research is typical when searching for a physician. When asked if the participant looked for a physician online, 61 percent (114) responded with "yes." Seventy-one percent (126) of the participants indicated that they viewed the physician profile information. More specifically, when asked if the participant ever viewed a video profile for any physician during the selection process, 24 percent (43) of the responses indicated that the participant viewed a video profile.

The participants were asked about whether or not a physician identifies as being accepting of LGBTQ patients is important. Sixty-seven percent (123) responded that it does matter to the participant that the doctor identifies as accepting. When asked why, participants provided responses such as, "I know I can easily talk freely without thinking about their reaction," or "less judgment of me and my lifestyle and hopefully, more focused on my health issue." Furthermore, one participant indicated, "Every little bit helps. If I worry that their care may be compromised by their judgment, I am not going to have faith in my medical care . . . that I am truly healthy. That nothing has been missed."

Participants were also asked whether or not they would be more likely to select a physician who identifies as either being LGBTQ or an ally. Eighty-nine percent (159) participants indicated increased probability of selecting a physician identified as an ally or LGBTQ. The participants mentioned being comfortable with an LGBTQ or ally physician. One participant stated, "because I would feel safer to be who I am." Another participant elegantly stated:

> It is more comforting to disclose information to someone you are comfortable with, someone who identifies with the same community, understands the dynamics of same-sex relationships and understands the overall background. It is always nicer to speak with someone who knows exactly where you are coming from and can relate to it. Not that I am uncomfortable with physicians who identify as heterosexual, I just believe if it came

down to both physicians having the same qualifications—I would choose the LBGTQ identifying physician.

DISCUSSION

Implications on Medical Practice

When comparing the current survey results of this study to the above-cited studies from the 1980s, prior to when the WHO declassified homosexuality as an illness in 1990, in some aspects, definite improvements become evident. For example, Johnson et al. (1981) found that 40 percent of lesbians thought that the quality of care would be negatively affected by the physician's knowledge of sexual orientation (p. 24) as compared to 11 percent in the current study. Johnson et al.'s study also found that only 18 percent of lesbian women disclosed sexual orientation to a physician (p. 23). The current study indicates a significantly higher level of disclosure at 72 percent for PCPs and 83 percent for OB/GYNs. These comparisons clearly demonstrate an improvement with increased open communication between WSW patients and physicians; however, the number of WSW failing to disclose to a PCP or OB/GYN is still too high, with approximately 25 percent still choosing not to disclose.

Johnson et al. (1981) discussed that several participants indicated that "a major hindrance to effective communication was the assumption by the physician that every patient is heterosexual" (p. 25). One respondent from the current study indicated the same: "There were already assumptions made about me by the physician, as usual when it comes to sexual orientation. Having to break through those assumptions can be uncomfortable for both parties."

The challenge for medical practice is that the current standardized procedures for medical practitioners involve heteronormative assumptions about behavior. The key piece to the solution is to rewrite the protocol and retrain the medical community in a new procedure that does not invoke those assumptions. A behavioral routine, which involves a set of diagnostic and interaction protocols that does not assume heterosexual practices by the patient, is needed to accommodate the diverse pool of patients. Providing a revised framework for standardized interaction procedures that permits persons to identify themselves with sexual orientations and practices without assuming heterosexuality is the first step.

A trend analysis that analyzes the medical literature by Snyder (2011) demonstrates a general lack of research related to general or common health topics for LGBT people. Although a fair amount of research relates to gay men, especially regarding sexually transmitted diseases such as HIV, little research so far focuses on WSW (Snyder, 2011). Even though WSW experience the same medical conditions faced by heterosexual women, though perhaps to varying degrees, physician knowledge of a patient's sexual orientation is critical not only for accurate diagnoses and treatment but also for creating a supportive and safe environment to foster effective communication between patient and doctor. Understanding a patient's sexual orientation is the first step for creating open and honest communication between the physician and the patient. Ultimately, this is absolutely required to ensure the patient's comfort, trust, and the highest quality of care.

In June 2013, the United States Supreme Court made a landmark ruling related to same-sex marriage that basically allowed for same-sex marriages, when obtained in states where same-sex marriage is legal, to be recognized by the federal government. Future studies should examine if being a WSW married to another woman increases or diminishes the rate in which people disclose sexual orientation to their physicians or exclude partners from health care experiences. Such studies should include participants in both states where same-sex marriage is legal and states where it is not to construct a comparison between the two samples.

Ultimately, respect and honesty lie at the heart of being able to safely disclose one's sexual orientation to a physician. As one participant simply responded, "It is important to be open and honest to doctors about your sexual practices so they can provide appropriate care, and appropriate routine testing can be done. Also I feel no shame for being who I am."

NOTE

1. A special thank you goes out to Dr. Mary Burke, MD, Assistant Clinical Professor of Obstetrics & Gynecology, Medical College of Wisconsin, whose commitment to offering compassionate quality care free of judgment and regardless of patient sexual orientation inspired this research.

Coming Out Conversations and Gay/ Bisexual Men's Sexual Health

A Constitutive Model Study

Jimmie Manning

"I thought my family would know me better. That this is the same person that they have loved for years. But they didn't. They just saw me as another stereotype. I was just, just another gay man who slept around and. And that's what they saw right then."

—Mark, 22

"You would think that if anyone knew not to ask those kinds of things, it would be my doctor. But no. There he was, acting like everything you hear about gay men is true. And from my experience it's not."

—Evan, 33

The epigraphs for this chapter come from two men who were interviewed for this research project.[1] Although they deal with interactions involving two different social identities (family members and health care providers, respectively), they help illustrate a recurring theme introduced by gay men who talked about their coming out experiences: a suspicion regarding sexual health that often seems to permeate coming out conversations. Of course, the context of coming out to a family member is much different than that of coming out to a health care provider. As the participants in this study note, coming out to a family member makes it feel as if more is at stake because of the enduring and highly personal nature of families. If there is rejection by a family member, that feels more important and more permanent than rejection from a health care provider. As one participant said, "You can always find a new doctor. Finding a new family member is a lot harder to do." Yet, at the same time, because a coming out conversation with a health care provider is articulated as less intimate—participants used terms such as "clinical" or "official" to describe these experiences—it does not mean that the implications of such conversations cannot have highly personal meanings. As one participant offered, "It hurt to hear him [the doctor] say it more than anyone else. Because he's educated on this stuff. He knows the research on a deeper level. And so if he still sees us [gay men] that way, that's a pretty good mark of how society sees us." Moreover, and as the data in this study reflect, those seeing health care professionals already feel vulnerable. Rejection based on sexual identity can make an already anxiety-inducing situation even scarier.

This chapter, then, focuses on coming out conversations between gay men and family members as well as between them and their health care providers. Both are presented with the goal of helping health care clinicians and other interested professionals to understand the coming out experiences of gay and bisexual men so that they can foster open lines of communication beyond the coming out conversation. Although it may seem curious to pair coming out disclosures in both family and health care contexts, the interview data used for this study will establish how the discourses are linked.

One immediate relationship between the two discourses is that coming out experiences with family members and health care providers were the only two contexts listed by those who participated in the study where questions about sexual health came up. In both contexts, even if the recipient of the coming out disclosure meant well by introducing sexual health, many times their statements or questions were not well received. This study looks across both of those experiences to examine how they might be interlinked and how each informs the other. Even though many people have wonderful and accepting coming out experiences, coming out can still be nerve-racking (Adams, 2011; Manning, 2014). Those in coming out conversations—both the person disclosing sexual orientation and the receiver of the coming out disclosure—are often highly sensitive about the moment and might be at a loss about what to say, how to offer support, how to acknowledge their feelings, or about communication during the conversation in general (Manning, 2014). These anxieties can cause or allow for emotional health concerns (Manning, 2014). However, as this chapter demonstrates, there is a possibility for those who are coming out to especially feel dehumanized when topics of sexual health are introduced by the receiver to sexual health conversations.

To unpack these experiences, this study begins by presenting a constitutive, theoretically inclusive model of coming out. This model helps to explain how lesbian, gay, and bisexual (LGB) people come to understand their non-heterosexual identity, how they go about communicating that identity with others, and how notions of coming out are culturally engrained. Special care is taken to point to how all three levels of this model tie into emotional, and sometimes physical, health.

A CONSTITUTIVE MODEL OF COMING OUT

Rust (2003) defines coming out as "the process by which individuals come to recognize that they have romantic or sexual feelings toward members of their own gender, adopt lesbian or gay (or bisexual) identities, and then share these identities with others" (p. 227). Research about coming out has happened primarily in three contexts. First, *sociopsychological studies* have helped to explain a person's cognitive understandings and emotions as they begin to realize and explore their nonheterosexual sexual identity. These studies include both a person's psychological identity development as well as the understandings they have about what it means to be LGB. Next, *cultural studies* have explored how cultures and societies make sense and react to nonheterosexual identities and behaviors. These studies look at social constructions of sex and sexuality as well as what Baxter (2011) would call *distal discourses*, or larger cultural discourses that people draw from when they interact with others. Finally, and most recently, *interactive studies* have started examining how people communicate sexual identity. That includes both their performances, or how they say and do things; as well as *proximal discourses*, or the things they actually say to other people. All three areas have yielded rich and useful findings that help both explain coming out in many different academic disciplines and professional study areas and explore coming out from a variety of epistemological stances. These three strands of coming out research are combined here in a *Constitutive Model of Coming Out* (figure 3.1) that illustrates the interplay of their different dimensions as they come together into a collective whole.

The Cognitive Level

At the center of this model is the *Cognitive Level* of coming out. This level draws primarily from the sociopsychological research and particularly explores how LGB individuals cognitively make sense of their nonheterosexual identity as well as the psychological effects resulting from their acceptance or rejection of it. The research in this area began with Cass's (1979, 1984) Homosexual Identity Formation Model (HIM). This model is widely cited and recognized. In fact, during the preparation of this chapter, twenty-three different guides, pamphlets, brochures, or websites were examined that offered information about coming out. They all pointed to HIM either explicity or indirectly by listing its various stages. HIM not only serves as the germinal and most largely recognized model involved with the coming out process (Rust, 2003), but it has also been the driving force for research about coming out in virtually all social scientific disciplines (Rust) This psychological model

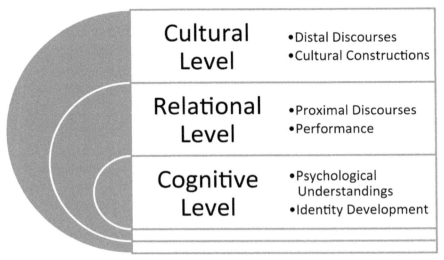

Figure 3.1.   Constitutive Model of Coming Out

examines the mental stages a LGB person goes through as he or she develops his or her understanding of self in terms of sexual orientation: Identity Confusion, Identity Comparison, Identity Tolerance, Identity Acceptance, Identity Pride, and Identity Synthesis (Cass, 1979; see table 3.1). These various stages are described as "goals" individuals strive toward "to acquire an identity of 'homosexual' fully integrated within the individual's overall concept of self" (Cass, 1979, p. 220). In other words, to find an adjusted sense of mental health, someone would need to go through all of the stages of the model.

As other researchers continued to explore coming out, they soon came to realize that HIM, although an excellent beginning model, was also entrenched in a rigid structure that did not necessarily allow for psychosocial differences in coming out experiences across cultures. An examination of some of the thought processes included in table 3.1 helps to illustrate this idea. Because of this, psychologists, sociologists, and sex scientists from other disciplines expanded on Cass's findings to develop more nuanced understandings. Troiden's (1988, 1989) research was the first notable extension of HIM, rejecting its linear stage by stage progression and arguing instead for a horizontal spiral where an individual could progress both up and down and back and forth across stages as she or he becomes more or less comfortable with certain elements of her or his own life and begins to accept or reject them. The model basically retains the essential elements of Cass's model, with the spiral element reflecting the struggles in moving forward and backward in the process. Similar to the Troiden model, but removed from the Cass foundation,

Table 3.1. Cass's (1979) Stages of Homosexual Identity Formation

Stage	Description	Representative Thought Process
Identity Confusion	Person begins to realize he or she has a nonheterosexual identity	"I think I might be gay."
Identity Comparison	Person begins to compare their sexual identity to his or her idea of heterosexuality	"It's going to be harder for me to have kids if I decide that I want them. Or get married."
Identity Tolerance	Person begins to present nonheterosexual identity to others	"I guess if I really am gay I should tell Andrea. She probably will be the most accepting."
Identity Acceptance	Person is more open to sharing identity and will begin to interact with other nonheterosexual people more frequently	"You know, hanging out with gay guys is a lot more fun than I thought it would be. I should introduce Andrea to the group."
Identity Pride	Person begins to enjoy, appreciate, or even celebrate nonheterosexual identity; a sense of "us versus them"	"Tomorrow is going to be so fun! My first gay bar! No dealing with boring straight people!"
Identity Synthesis	Person begins to see the commonality of their identity and the identities of others and as part of an integrated romantic and sexual world	"I don't think I ever want to get married, but I would like to be in a nice partnered relationship and maybe live in the 'burbs."

is D'Augelli's (1994) life span approach to sexual orientation identity development. This model emphasizes six developmental areas in sexual orientation that occur throughout life: exiting heterosexual identity, developing a personal gay identity status, developing a gay social identity, becoming a gay offspring, developing a gay intimacy status, and entering a gay community. Key to this model is the notion of "developmental plasticity" (p. 320), the way one must spontaneously respond to environmental factors or stimuli (D'Augelli, 1994). Also key is "interindividual differences" (p. 321) highlighting the distinctive developmental circumstances for an individual person based on sexual identity (D'Augelli, 1994).

As helpful as these models were for helping to identify and explore cognitive aspects of sexual identity, they also received criticism for their lack of cultural awareness and for retaining such a strong focus on the individual. Many of the studies ignored racial and ethnic considerations of coming out (Chan, 1995; Gonzales & Espin, 1996; Greene, 1994; Loiacano, 1989), asserted a hegemonic whiteness (Rosario, Schrimshaw, Hunter, & Braun, 2006), or undermined bisexuality (Rust, 1996), thus suggesting a need for a diverse sample of research participants. Finally, critiques suggest that many cognitive coming out models are often flawed because they almost always place a single person into the core of the analysis, allowing culture, community, and especially communicative relationships to be ignored or minimized in developing coming out scholarship (Diamond, 2003; Peplau & Garnets, 2000). Research continues in the cognitive realm, however, and is being supplemented by a rich body of research exploring cultural and relational dimensions of coming out.

The Cultural Level

The outer edge of the constitutive model represents the *Cultural Level* of coming out. It engulfs both inner levels for two reasons. First, a culture will almost certainly have an impact on the relationships and individuals in it. Within a given culture, identities and relationships are defined, rewarded, controlled, limited, or otherwise negotiated. As such, a person's cognitive and communicative abilities or understandings will be impacted by the cultures that surround and make intelligible what identities and relationships mean. Second, and in line with the first point, because cultures form the very notions of *sexual identity, sexual orientation, coming out,* or other related terms, and given that cultures are malleable and able to be changed, cultural understandings come into play with how a person's identities and relationships are communicated and psychologically processed. In other words, and in drawing from notions of constitutive theorizing (Baxter, 2004; Manning, 2014), interaction constitutes or creates social worlds. Observing both these constructions and how they are being constructed, then, allows for very real understandings of things that are not always physically tangible. For example, a concept such as the closet is one that is not literal—it cannot be touched, smelled, tasted, or physically handled—but rather is one that exists because people interacting agree, on some level, that it exists. That does not mean that the closet does not have profound effects upon those who experience it. Rather, it suggests that social interaction is what creates a notion of the closet.

　　Many scholars have explored constructions of the closet, but the most recognized and cited of these articulations is Sedgwick's (1990) epistemological interrogation of the closet. Published as the now-classic *Epistemology of the Closet*, the book, which is an exercise in literary criticism that analyzes texts from well-known writers such as Melville or Proust, especially focuses on how binary oppositions of *homo* and *hetero* make sexuality much too simplified. As Sedgwick asserts, "Virtually any aspect of modern Western culture must be, not merely complete, but damaged in its central substance to the degree that it does not incorporate a critical analysis of modern homo/heterosexual definition" (1990, p. 1). In Sedgwick's view, matters of sexuality are negotiable but culturally embedded, and as such what is closeted and uncloseted is negotiable as well. That is, if someone is to come out of the closet, what does that mean? Can one really uncloset all of their sexuality? Even if someone acknowledges a socially labeled sexual identity, what does that really tell about who they are as a sexual being? Sedgwick's analysis also leads to questions about whether aspects of identity other than sexuality can be closeted. Those questions are certainly worthy of exploration.

Although Sedgwick's work was largely grounded in literary criticism, it has inspired the research of many who explore coming out at the Cultural Level by using ethnographic or other qualitative approaches. For example, Adams (2011) drew from Sedgwick (1990) to describe ways, or *situational paradoxes*, that allow for confusion or frustration for nonheterosexual people. Most of these paradoxes put blame on the person coming out, whether that be for coming out too early or too soon, to one person before another, or even for being nervous about revealing sexual identity. In reflecting on these paradoxes, he notes that,

> Paradox occurs when a person with same-sex attraction is held accountable—by self and others—for taking a wrong course of action, making the wrong move: there are consequences for a person who comes out or does not, who comes out too soon or not soon enough, who completes the coming-out process or finds completion impossible, or who comes out most of the time, some of the time, or never at all (Adams, 2011, p. 112).

As Adams's work demonstrates, work at the Cultural Level helps to make evident how cultures situate people and identities. Other scholars who have explored how coming out is facilitated or informed by culture include Bacon (1998) who enacted a language-oriented study of coming out, later extended by Tawake (2006), that positions coming out narratives as a cultural form of rhetoric aimed toward a queer movement of liberation.

As that all implies, the Cultural Level also includes the political implications associated with coming out and LGB identity in general. Observations made at the Cultural Level point to some of the ways that sexuality can be constructed in contemporary culture. Unlike the Cognitive Level, where findings are based more on an individual's psychological response, the Cultural Level tends to explore how meaning circulates throughout a culture. That means media representations, public law and policy, organizational rules, and any other intelligible aspect of a culture will play into individuals' and societies' understandings of coming out. These understandings are often negotiated with other members of a culture at the Relational Level.

The Relational Level

Recently, scholars have begun to explore the interpersonal disclosures that occur as part of coming out. Coming out, in the communicative sense, is not isolated from the individuals who are sharing or receiving coming out disclosures; nor are they separated from the cultures that inform, surround, and otherwise make intelligible what it means to come out. As such, the Relational Level is nestled between the cultural and cognitive levels of the model. The Relational Level focuses on coming out as it occurs in interpersonal relationships. Specifically, it explores *proximal discourses*, or the things people say directly to each other as they relate to coming out. Those proximal discourses will draw from *distal discourses*, or the elements of culture that allow a coming out disclosure to be understood. So, for instance, if someone says, "I'm gay," that proximal disclosure ties into a larger, distal idea of "coming out." Depending on an individual's experiences and ideas about coming out, he or she will respond with another proximal utterance that draws from a distal discourse. That could be, "You know it's an abomination" (drawing from a distal discourse of religion), "God made you perfectly, and if that's gay then so be it" (drawing from a different distal discourse of religion), "But you don't act gay!" (drawing from a distal discourse that suggests LGB people behave a particular way), or, as was common for the participants of this study, "Are you being careful sexually?" (drawing from a distal discourse that gay or bisexual men are at risk to contract sexually transmitted diseases or infections). These notions of proximal and distal discourses are developed from a line of theorizing that communication theorist Leslie A. Baxter refers to as the second iteration of Relational Dialectical Theory (Baxter, 2011).

Many of the studies at the Relational Level came later than studies explored in the Cognitive or Cultural Levels, as they were often in response to critiques of those two areas that assumed how communication would occur between people based on psychological or cultural indicators. Plummer (1995) was among the first to interrogate those assumptions, exploring how people tell their sexual stories, including stories of coming out. Later, scholars explored coming out as a performative act that has implications for both the speaker and hearer (e.g., Chirrey, 2003; Speer & Potter, 2000). These studies, situated in the Cultural Level, began to point to the importance of exploring coming out interactions. On the Cognitive front, studies began to explore the impacts of coming out on an individual level as they related to others. These include studies exploring psychological processes leading to decisions to disclose sexual orientation (e.g., Franke & Leary, 1991; Griffith & Hebl, 2002); the consequences or effects of such a disclosure with family members (e.g., Cramer & Roach, 1988; Schope, 2002); or effects of coming out in the workplace (King, Reilly, & Hebl, 2008; Russ, Simonds, & Hunt, 2002).

A different, but related, body of relational coming out research has focused more on coming out conversations and the types of interaction that occurs when a person reveals his or her sexual identity to another. For example, narratives of coming out conversations were used to develop a typology of six salient and nonexclusive ways (meaning a single conversation could fall into multiple conversation types) coming out conversations tend to occur: as pre-planned, emergent, coaxed, forced, romantic, or educational/activist (Manning, in press; see table 3.2).

Regardless of conversation type, and as one might expect, coming out conversations tend to follow a particular format (Manning, 2006). They usually begin with an introduction, prefacing that an important, perhaps life-changing conversation, is taking place. Introductions can be quite short ("Mom, do you have a minute? There's something we need to talk about."), but they can also be longer and involve a story or narrative to introduce the idea that the conversation will be about sexual orientation. The introduction can also be from the receiver of the coming out disclosure, as he or she might hint or even forcefully demand that someone should come out (as is demonstrated in the typology). In professional situations, such as a conversation with a health care provider, it is quite possible that an introduction as presented in this trajectory will not exist.

For most conversations, however, after the introduction a disclosure is made. These are often direct ("I'm gay."), but they can also be indirect or ambiguous ("And so I think now, I might start dating other women."). That leads to the reaction period, where questions or comments about the disclosure are discussed (and that the data about families presented in this study largely explores). Finally, closing statements are made that usually contain some sort of indication as to where the parties stand, where the relationship might be going, and that often include particularly memorable messages for both the person disclosing and the receiver. These four elements of a coming out conversation (the introduction, disclosure, reaction, and close) are not normative in the sense that they suggest what *should* happen in a conversation, but rather offer a trajectory of what one might expect if they are involved with a discursive coming out experience.

Table 3.2. Manning's (in press) Nonexclusive Typology of Coming Out Conversations

Conversation Type	Defined	Representative Dialogue
Pre-planned	An LGB person decides he or she is going to come out to another in advance and prepares accordingly	Arturo: Mom, the reason I invited you here to have dinner tonight is because there is something I want to share with you.
Emergent	An LGB person sees an opportunity to introduce her or his sexual and romantic identity into conversation and takes it	Abuela: I just saw on the news what is happening in Russia with gay and lesbian people. It is disgusting to see people being treated so poorly! We are all God's people. Arturo: You know, Abuela, I'm glad to hear you say that. There's something I've been meaning to share with you for a while now, but I wasn't sure how to bring it up.
Coaxed	An LGB person is encouraged to share his or her sexual and romantic identity	Juan: You know, brother, there is nothing you cannot tell me. Arturo: I know that, Juan. Juan: I want us to be close, and that means sharing everything about our lives—including who we love.
Forced	A person demands that an LGB person share her or his sexual identity	Lucy: You keep telling me you aren't interested in dating right now, but I know what's up. Tell me, Arturo, or I'll tell everyone and shame you in front of our whole high school!
Romantic	An LGB person comes out through romantic or sexual advances	Miguel: Oh, I've had too much to drink tonight, my friend. Arturo: Me too. Maybe that's why I've got the courage to finally tell you how I feel about you after all of these years.
Educational/ Activist	An LGB person comes out, usually to an audience of people, as a means of educating or encouraging others	Arturo: I thank you all for inviting me to speak to your group today. Before I begin, however, I believe it is important that you know my perspective is one that is informed by my sexual identity.

EXTENDING THE RELATIONAL LEVEL: FAMILIES AND HEALTH CARE PROVIDERS

The study presented in this chapter is situated in the Relational Level and moves toward ideas of what might ought to happen in order to create open, affirming coming out conversations. It extends existing work about coming out conversations (Manning, 2006, 2014, in press) to explore how interactions are occurring between gay and bisexual men and their families as well as between them and their health care providers in coming out conversations where topics of sexual health are introduced. Specifically, it expands on a finding noted by Manning (2014) regarding a theme found in the initial coding of his data, "frustration with concerns about sexual health," that saturated for men but not for women. That men articulated this experience in their narratives of coming out conversations, whereas women did not, was notable in and of itself. However, it also points to an underexplored area of health communication research regarding gay or bisexual men and health care providers. Studies of lesbian interaction with medical professionals abound, mostly from the 1990s. Eliason and Schope (2001) suggest that this attention paid to lesbian health issues might be because many studies about gay male health were directed toward HIV/AIDS treatment and practices; therefore, the body of research exploring lesbian health care needs served as a way of supplementing the large amount of attention paid to gay and bisexual men. Additionally, because so much research about men who have sex with men was aimed at HIV/AIDS prevention, other avenues of inquiry were not explored.

Many concerns shared by lesbian participants in those studies add to the context of this study. For example, lesbian women often complain that they receive counseling or education about inappropriate or unnecessary issues such as reproductive health (Lehmann, Lehmann, & Kelly, 1998). That mirrors data in this study that shows many times gay men felt the counseling or advice they received was unneeded or unwarranted. The education lesbian participants reported might have been a result of heteronormative assumption, where a physician or other health care provider assumed the female patient as heterosexual (Lehmann, Lehmann, & Kelly, 1998). As that suggests, many health care providers do not inquire about sexual orientation, and lesbian women report that they do not come out on their own, either. In one study, 60 percent of the women surveyed were out to their parents, but only 31 percent were out to their physician (Lehmann, Lehmann, & Kelly, 1998). Hitchcock and Wilson (1992) found evidence that when lesbians do come out, it is often only after trust is established with a health care provider, and that can be long into the relationship. Lesbian women in rural communities might especially feel apprehension, as many report they are concerned that their sexual identity could be leaked by a health care provider and so they are reluctant to share it (Tiemann, Kennedy, & Haga, 1998). These findings are in harmony with the data collected and analyzed for this study, and they add context to the larger picture of LGB sexual health.

METHODS

The data used in this manuscript come from a larger qualitative research study exploring coming out narratives provided by 182 gay, lesbian, and bisexual participants. Thirty participants were individually asked to share the stories of their most recent and a most memorable coming out experiences in an interview session. After each narrative was provided, participants were asked to consider both the positive and negative communicative elements. An additional 130 participants also provided two coming out narratives through an open-ended online survey, again identifying positive and negative communicative elements of those experiences. Finally, in response to mentions of sexual health in the original data, twenty-two additional gay and bisexual men were recruited and interviewed to talk about coming out experiences with physicians.

Participants for the study were located through snowball sampling (Manning & Kunkel, 2014), beginning with seven online groups centered around discussion of LGB issues. Fifteen men and fifteen women provided the interviews. Of the 130 participants responding to the survey, sixty-two identified as men, sixty-seven as women, and four of the participants also identified as transgender. One person refused to identify in terms of sex. Those being interviewed about their health care experiences were all biologically male and identified as men, with eighteen identifying as gay and four identifying as bisexual. The participants ranged in age from eighteen to seventy-two years old, with a mean age of 31.4 years. The participants were racially and ethnically diverse, with white, non-Hispanic participants only making up 65 percent of the sample.

For the purposes of this study, only interviews and surveys with more than a passing mention of sexual health were included; and then only those for participants who identified as men. That led to data from thirty-five diverse participants and featuring seventy coming out narratives. Ultimately, initial interview transcripts, completed surveys, and follow-up interview transcripts allowed for three forms of data that could be analyzed using a multiadic approach (Manning, 2013). This multiadic approach allowed participants both the freedom to tell their often unheard stories (Manning, 2010) while simultaneously serving as a triangulated form of data collection to ensure valid results (Manning & Kunkel, 2014).

Data Analysis

The multiadic data set was initially explored using a standard thematic analysis approach (Braun & Clarke, 2006). After initial themes were developed and considered, two additional forms of analysis were enacted. First, a modified version of Spradley's (1979) semantic coding was applied, specifically Manning and Kunkel's (2014) approach to taxonomic development. The goal of this taxonomic development is to create categories that describe specific types of or possibilities for communication. For this study, that meant a list of salient possibilities or ways sexual health was introduced in coming out conversations. Second, to draw comparisons and contrasts across the two cases (family contexts and health care contexts) and to explore for contradictions within each of the two cases, Baxter's (2011) contrapuntal analysis was applied. Contrapuntal analysis is intimately tied to Relational Dialectical Theory and involves examining themes or discourses and examining where they compete, contradict, or otherwise come into tension. Attention was especially paid to where family, health care, and invoked distal/cultural discourses came into interplay. That is, even though families and health institutions will certainly add to ideas of what it means to come out as well as what it means to be LGB, they are only but two systems of discourse that play into a larger social discourse of what it means to come out. Yet, at the same time, the focus of this study also allows for discourses in each of the domains, families and health care, to be considered in comparison to and as they might help to build each other. How this analysis functions will become more apparent as results and data exemplars are presented and explained.

RESULTS

The results of the analysis are presented here in each contextual domain, beginning with family coming out experiences and then moving into health care domains.

Families Expressing Concerns about Sexual Health

The taxonomic coding allowed for the development of a typology showing three ways sexual health was introduced in coming out conversations with family members: most often as an *added thought*, which was viewed as caring; sometimes as a *central concern*, which was viewed as negative; and, for a couple of participants, as an *irrational sidebar*, which was viewed as negative and hopeless.

Sexual health as added thought. In many cases, family members introduced sexual health as an added thought during the conversation, often toward the end. As one man shared about his sister, "She then told me, 'I have to say it, I know you are probably safe but be careful. It can be a dangerous sexual world out there." He later acknowledged, "I know she told me to do that because she cared. It represented the love she felt for me and that she wanted the best for my life." Another gay man shared, "After it was done, they hugged me and my dad joked, 'I don't know how to give you the same sex talk for this, but you do know to be safe right?'" When asked about this interaction in a member check interview, the participant shared, "The way he did it was kind of nice. It kind of said, 'I don't know if I get what it means to be gay, but I'm trying.' And introduced in that context, it was a nice way to let me know that he still had my best interests at heart." As these examples demonstrate, mentioning sexual health as a side thought in the overall coming out conversation was often not seen as a negative thing. On the contrary, participants indicated that it showed positive concern.

A notable exception to this positivity was mentioned by two participants who said a parent mentioned HIV/AIDS by name. In one case, the participant was upset because his mother mentioned that she would always have to be concerned about HIV and AIDS. As he shares,

> It was all fine, pretty boring actually, and then out of nowhere, toward the end, she goes, "And now I have to worry about whether or not you're going to get AIDS, but I'll get over it." I kind of stopped, but my back was turned to her so I don't know if she noticed or not. But then I just went up the stairs and to my room and I cried. Out of all of it, that hurt the most . . . She was saying I was a burden. That now I was just something scary to her that she had to think about. And like she wanted to say more, but was resisting, and just had to get that in.

Another participant shared a story about his father, writing, "At the end my mom asked my dad if he had anything to say. And he goes, 'You know most gay men get AIDS. I expect you to not be one of them.' It was cold and monotone. I almost wish he would have said nothing at all." In this instance, the participant was coming out to his mother and father together, and although his mother talked quite a bit, his father was silent except for that utterance.

Sexual health as central concern. For many family members, mostly parents, sexual health was mentioned as a central concern in coming out conversations. As one man described in telling about coming out to his parents, "My mother didn't say anything for about five minutes. She just cried. My dad sat there looking down. Then when my mom finally talked, she said, 'now I'm scared. You know, most gay men get AIDS. I don't want that for you.'" Later in his narrative, the participant expressed how his mother's worry seemed genuine but created a situation where he felt he needed to take care of her and make sure that she was OK in the interaction. He also regretted that "virtually the whole thing was about AIDS and sex." Although most of the parents described their parents as heartbroken or even angry about the possibility of the contraction of AIDS or other diseases, some mentioned that things were stated more matter-of-factly. As one participant wrote, "She said she knew already, then she gave me a lecture on safe sex." When asked about the lecture in a follow-up interview, the participant noted, "I guess the more I think about it all, the more it is funny to me. Coming out is more than about being sexual, but that is what people think about. So I think that is why she decided then was the time to give me 'the talk.' And that was about all the conversation was."

Despite the matter-of-fact nature of the talk, this participant still, like all of the participants who mentioned these experiences, saw the discussion of sexual health as negative. As he shared, "I know it was an easy thing for her to jump to and discuss, because she follows all of the safe sex and other health stuff. But I was hoping for more emotional stuff and questions about how happy I am. We're talking about my love life, not just my sex life." Other participants agreed. "I didn't come out to my dad just to hear him lecture me on AIDS for an hour," one gay man said. A bisexual man shared, "Every time I thought we would move on to another topic, they kept going back to how dangerous gay sex was and how I had to be careful." Another gay man said that he came out to both of his parents separately and received a similar response both times: "I was worried about hearing about religion. Instead I got a lecture on gay sex. It made me wish I never told them." As these exemplars demonstrate, topics of sexual health dominating coming out conversations were not appreciated.

Sexual health as irrational sidebar. Though it was rare, some mentioned that—especially in the case of a coming out conversation where disclosure was not well received—a parent or sibling brought up sexual health in an aggressive or highly dramatic way. As one participant shared in his narrative,

> She said she was going to be supportive, and she said that we should keep it from my dad for now. Then I went to hug her, and she held her hand up, and I said "I thought you were going to be supportive." She started saying, "I think we should go and have you tested." I told her that I was not sexually active and I did not even have a boyfriend and everything I told her she kept repeating, "I think we should go and have you tested." Then she started crying and yelling things about AIDS and gay men not controlling their sex and that I needed to get in the habit now. Then she

said it was not me being gay that was bad but the "gay lifestyle" was and
that she had to protect me from it.

This participant's written narrative demonstrates how some recipients of coming out disclosures mention two aspects of a person: his or her nonheterosexual
identity, and then some aspect of who the person truly is. That consideration
is important to considering the tensions between loving and stereotyping expressed by participants.

   **Contradicting discourses in families: loving versus stereotyp-
ing.** In the case of gay and bisexual men, constructions of nonheterosexual
identity frequently include ideas of promiscuity that are almost always
framed as a health risk, or the listing of health risks, especially HIV or AIDS,
that are mentioned without any explicit link to promiscuity, but where participants felt it was implied. In fact, during interviews many of the men made
it clear that their parents tried to not point at them as being promiscuous,
but rather as gay men in general. As one man stated, "She [my mother] said
it wasn't me she was worried about, but you never knew about other gay
men." Another shared, "My sister said that there were lots of sickos who
were gay because their family didn't accept it, and so they did dangerous
things, and that I had to be careful." At the same time, participants rejected
this pathologizing of other gay men and saw it as more of a reflection of who
they are. As one man shared, "OK, so you can say all you want that it's not
what I do that worries you, but if you're afraid I'm going to get AIDS, then
yeah, you are worried that I'm like the other guys. Because you've already
said that's why they get it." As another participant succinctly put it, "Basically, they [my family] see me as a stereotype. They didn't put it that way,
but when half of what they're saying is about sleeping around and catching
diseases, then that's how they're seeing me then."

   This frustration played into a commonly expressed tension for the gay
and bisexual men of *being seen as the family member they love* and *being seen as
a stereotype* by their family members. The push and pull of that experience
was important in their narratives and their overall evaluation of the coming
out conversation. When sexual health was brought up as an added thought
in coming out conversations, the men reported that it showed caring and
concern. When it became the main topic of the conversation or used as an
attack point, that made them feel more like they were not being viewed as
a person but more as a stereotypical gay man. It is important to note that
those who said it was brought up in the coming out conversation stated that
it continued to come up in future conversations about their sexual identity.
"My mom doesn't like to talk about it at all," one man shared, "but when

she does, it is always about me making sure to be safe and to avoid men on the Internet." He and other men frequently expressed that this made them feel as if being gay were only about sexual aspects and not romantic aspects of the identity. "Not once have they asked me about dating or a boyfriend," a participant said. "Instead, it is always about being safe. Little do they know I'm more likely to have a broken heart than an STD with how my love life goes."

Health Care Providers Expressing Concerns about Sexual Health

The taxonomic analysis reviewed three ways sexual health was introduced in conversations with health care providers: as a *routine question*, which was usually reviewed as positive; as an *act of suspicion*, which was reviewed as negative; and as a *nerve-racking experience*, which was viewed as negative and incompetent. Negative case analysis is also provided for the health care provider taxonomy, as two participants explained they did not reveal their sexual orientation to a health care provider. One participant explained he was afraid his health care provider would tell his parents; and the other because he felt it was none of his health care provider's business.

Sexual health as routine question. In interviewing the participants for this study, all but two said they came out to a physician during a routine question, or, in some cases, when the physician asked a heteronormative question and they felt as if they did not want to lead the physician down a wrong path. When it was mentioned in a routine or matter-of-fact way, this made patients feel better. "My doctor asked me if I was sexually active, and I said yes," one participant shared. "And then he asked me if there was anything he should know about my sex life or if I had any questions, and I said, 'Well, I'm gay.' And he goes, 'Thanks for telling me. Anything else?' and then that was that." When asked why that made him feel comfortable, he responded, "Because he was cool about it. So I thought, well, if I ever have any issues I don't think he'll be judgmental or grossed out."

Similar stories involved correcting a doctor when he or she mistakenly identified the participant as heterosexual. "My doctor goes, 'So you do you have a girlfriend?' when she was asking me all the medical questions, and I go, 'No, but I have a boyfriend.' And she just smiled and joked about putting her foot in her mouth. I told her not to worry about it." When asked why that situation made him comfortable, he responded, "Because she admitted right up front it was insensitive, what she did, but she didn't make a big deal out of it." Unfortunately, quite a few participants shared experiences where a "big deal" was made.

Sexual health as act of suspicion. When asked about his most recent coming out experience, a participant shared a written narrative that included the following:

> The most recent experience I had coming out to someone was my doctor. He has been the family doctor for a long time, so he has basically seen me grow into the man I am today. When I went to see him, I was already embarrassed because of the reason I was there. I know now that what I had was a hemorrhoid, and that my father who has never had sex with a man started getting them in his twenties to. I had anal sex where I received it for the first time just a week before I got one, so I didn't know what was wrong and thought it was because of that. My boyfriend told me it wasn't because he had let me give it to him many times and it never happened to him. I thought I should check to make sure. When I told the doctor this story, all he did was lecture me about how dangerous gay sex is and making sure I had condoms and telling me that it really was not a good practice. Then he told me that I should reconsider my activities before I get in some real trouble. I was embarrassed and humiliated and I have not gone back to the doctor since. To tell you the truth I believe he probably doesn't care.

The narrative speaks for itself in terms of why the participant saw the interaction as a negative one. The suspicious reaction of the physician created a situation where open communication could not continue and the doctor-patient relationship was terminated. When asked about how this situation might have impacted other relationships, he shared:

> The next doctor I went to, I was scared to tell her. And I made sure it was a woman, because I thought she might be more open minded. But I told her and told her about the problem and she told me it may be that the sex helped it along, but that most people don't get a hemorrhoid from having anal sex. I never got that with my family's doctor because all he was worried about was me getting worse things than a hemorrhoid.

In interviewing participants for this portion of the study, many other stories of suspicion were shared. Some said their doctors seemed suspicious of whether or not they were telling the truth about their sexual activity. As one interview exchange progressed:

Participant: He looked at me and goes, "You really only had three partners? Ever?" Now what man do you know to lie about sex?

Jimmie: Well—

Participant: Scratch that. That's the problem. Straight men can have all the sex they want, and it's great. Gay men do it, and we're whores.

Jimmie: So do you think that's how the doctor saw you?

Participant: As a whore?

Jimmie: Well, yeah.

Participant: No doubt. Every time I go to him, he reminds me of my sexual health and asks me if I need condoms. Bitch didn't do that once when he thought I was straight.

Similar stories were shared where the physician would suggest an HIV/AIDS test, or in other cases, as one participant called it, "a full battery of STD tests." One participant complained because his doctor kept insisting that he was bottoming during sex. "I don't even bottom, but he kept telling me that it was OK because he knew gay men do that. They do, but I haven't."

Sexual health as a nerve-racking experience. A third approach mentioned by participants involved physicians acting nervous. "He was literally shaking, like the clipboard was moving," one participant shared. "When I told him that I was gay, he stopped asking all the sex questions he used to ask at my annual physical," said another participant. "He just looks at the questions, and then kind of pauses, and then moves on." Some participants shared that their physicians tried to engage conversation about sex, but that it was awkward. As one interviewee narrated:

So I go, "No, no. You should know I'm gay." And he goes, "Oh. OK. Well, that's a perfectly acceptable answer. Congrats on that!" And I thought in my head, "Did he just congratulate me for being gay?" And it must've shown on my face because then he goes, "Sorry. I guess that's kind of a strange response. I was just trying to be affirming." But the way he said it, it was almost like a robot. I mean, it was nice and all. He was really trying. But it was so... awkward. Especially because I was half naked.

Concerns about stigma and privacy. As mentioned, two participants in the interview sessions mentioned they did not come out to their physicians. One participant said it was because of his concerns that his physician would stigmatize his sexual identity:

Participant: He doesn't seem like the kind of man who wants to hear that his patient is gay.

Jimmie: Tell me about that.

Participant: I think, uh, it is a lot of how he acts.

Jimmie: Mmhmm.

Participant: And, when you go to his office, it is decorated with crosses and other religious stuff. And, uh, the magazines, they all are religious, too. So I don't really get the feeling, or it doesn't seem like he would be comfortable hearing it.

Jimmie: So the way the office is decorated is part of what deters you?

Participant: Yeah. There's Bible verses and everything.

As can be seen from the participant's description, he avoids coming out to his health care provider because he is nervous that religious dogma might prevent that provider from being accepting. In his explanation, he draws from a common cultural discourse that those who display their Christianity in public ways are likely to reject nonheterosexual people.

The other participant saw it as none of his physician's business. "Sex is private," he said, "and unless I have a disease or need help, then he doesn't need to know." When asked about sexual health needs, he responded that he was safe and so he was not in need of a physician's care. "In college every semester in the pride alliance they gave us a safe sex talk," he said. When asked how he responds to questions about sex from his physician, he replied, "Like I said, doctors don't really need to know about your sex life unless something is wrong. And that will not apply to me. When they ask those questions, I refuse to answer."

Contradicting discourses in health care conversations: individuality versus deviancy. Using contrapuntal analysis to examine conflicting themes revealed that many times those coming out to health care providers experienced a tension between discourses of their *individual identities as people* and their *deviancy as connected to minoritized sexual identity*. Easily the most dominant theme that illustrates this discursive tension involved health care provider suspicion of the possibility of committed and monogamous relationships. Participant narratives such as this one were not uncommon:

> I told him no, I was gay. After that he asked me if I was sexually active. I said yes. He asked me if I was safe. I told him yes. He asked me what that meant, and I told him that me and my partner after being together for two years had been tested three times in a year's time and were negative, and so we stopped using condoms. Well, that was the end of it. He would not hear of it. He told me that gay men could never have that "luxury" and that we had to be extra careful. I told him I trusted my partner, and he said something along the lines of "well, I hope you trust him with your life." I was offended. I know me and my partner are remaining faithful.

As the close of that excerpt reflects, the cultural stereotype of promiscuous gay men is in tension with the identity of the couple.

Even for those participants who were not partnered were frustrated by the messages regarding monogamy they received. "My doctor asked me if I was sexually active, and I said yes," one man shared as part of his coming out conversation narrative. "Then he asked me how many partners I had in the last year. I told him one. He goes, 'Are you sure?' I said yes. And he goes, 'You know what you tell me is confidential.' I was angry." Once again, a tension between socially constructed gay behavior comes into conflict with the provider-patient relationship. Some participants speculated this kind of behavior could result from doctors not actually knowing any gay men. As one especially frustrated participant shared:

> He started asking me about my sex life, whether I had done it and all that. I told him, yes, yes, I have. And then he started talking about anal sex like he was reading it out of a dictionary or something, only a really boring dictionary that uses lots of words. I finally stopped him and said, "Yes, I know what it is. I've done it plenty of times." He then started telling me how tender the ass tissue is, only in doctor words, and I was looking at him the whole time thinking, "Has this guy ever talked to a gay guy before?" I feel sorry for the kid who just came out of the closet who has to listen to this guy. He doesn't know shit about anal sex!

This participant, like many others, suspected that his health care provider did not know gay men, but, as he framed it, "Kind of a medical diagram of what a gay man is supposed to be. Which doesn't get at half the story."

Just as with the family interviews, participants also reported frustration with being asked about being tested for HIV by their health care providers. "It is insulting that they would do that," one participant shared. "It's like they assume every gay men is doing something that means he should be tested." Another participant was frustrated that questions about HIV testing were asked even after his physician had screened for other risky behaviors. As he shared, "He went down a list, asking me if I had sex, with who, if I'm being safe. And then after all of that he still asked me if I wanted an HIV test. I told him I didn't need one, but he told me he thought it would be OK. I have a strong suspicion he only did that because I'm gay."

Connecting Discourses: Distal Stereotypes in Proximal Context

At first glance, it might appear that there is no relation between the two typologies of how sexual health is introduced in coming out conversations with family members or health care professionals. On one hand, and as alluded to at the beginning of the essay, family relationships are often highly personal, and the communication that happens within families, as well as the cultural com-munication that constitutes notions of what families are, is steeped in rituals, rules, and emotional expectations (Caughlin, Koerner, Schrodt, & Fitzpatrick, 2011). On the other hand, communication with health care providers is of-ten constructed—sometimes fairly and sometimes unfairly—as being rather anonymous and even depersonalized. In some ways, this makes sense as the relationships between patients and providers are often limited both by inter-personal time available to develop a relationship (Roter & Hall, 2006) as well as the implicit rules of privacy that tend to govern patient-provider interaction (Petronio & Sargent, 2011). Although this can be problematic in many con-texts beyond LGB care, as Stevens (1995) implies it is particularly problematic in situations such as patient-provider interaction with LGB individuals who find themselves immersed in a history of both distal and proximal discourses steeped in assuming, stigmatizing, or insensitive interaction. As the data reflect, however, these same negative and dehumanizing aspects of cultural construc-tions of same sex attraction can still be invoked in coming out conversations with family members—family members who have had the time and interac-tion to better know the person coming out.

Moreover, participants articulated connections between the conversa-tions happening with health care providers and conversations happening with family members; this illustrates how these discourses act not in isolation but in an interplay with each other. As one man explained, "After I came out to my doctor, and he seemed nervous about it, I decided not to come out to my family. If he could not handle it, I expect that they could not handle it either." Another was worried about privacy. "I still haven't come out to my parents, but I hope I will some day. But that means not coming out to my doctor, because if he told them that would be a huge mess." Other men talked directly about how one conversation influenced another. As one man said, "Coming out to my doctor made it easier to come out to my parents. I was now armed with facts I could use if they had concerns." Another shared, "After my parents accepted me, I was empowered. It made coming out to my doctor who goes to our church and is very religious a lot easier. Who cares what he thought?" Still, others reported that even with accepting parents they were afraid to come out to a health care provider, just as those who had an affirming experience with a health care provider reported they did not come out to one or more parents.

This notion that coming out experiences with health care providers plays into coming out experiences with family members and vice versa can be related to knowing or not knowing the individual who will receive the dis-closure. For example, if two parents continuously talked about "the disgusting and perverted social illness of homosexuality," that proximal discourse might make it to where their child refuses to come out. This study's data also help present the idea that there are also what I call *discursive specters*, or experiences that come with one discourse or interaction that encourage or discourage a person from engaging it in another time and place. For instance, the participant who said his doctor rejected him decided not to come out to his parents because, as he noted, if his "educated" health care professional who "knows the research on a deeper level" was rejecting him, he could not expect his parents to be accepting. Based on his interaction with this father, he was enacting segmentation (Baxter, 2011), or the purposeful avoidance of a discursive interaction because one knows that introducing a particular discourse—in this case same-sex attraction—could lead to conflict.

Yet those who received affirmation and affection often reported the situation as empowering, and that in later conversations where the reception was not so well-received the remnants of those past acceptances lingered and allowed the situation to be less stressful. That is, the discursive specter of where the discourse had successfully been previously remained in a future conversation. Those in coming out conversations should consider how their interaction is not but one conversation but rather another link in an on-going chain of discourse—and how that link in the discourse is negotiated can have an effect on future links. Moreover, if one is trying to be caring and conscientious in a coming out situation, the person coming out might not be ready to receive this love and support because a negative discursive specter is at play from earlier in the discursive chain. Given the tensions that can arise when sexual health is introduced to coming out conversations, it is important to consider how to talk about sexual health in ways where segmentation can be avoided and positive discursive specters constructed.

DISCUSSION

This study presents some strong considerations for how those who might receive a coming out disclosure should respond. Given the openness of many cultures that continue to decline in homohostility (Manning, 2009; Kaufman & Johnson, 2004), it is hard to imagine that most people will not have someone come out to them during their lifetimes. The data explored here through a lens of constitutive pragmatism, or the blending of various research findings across paradigm and tradition, offer some insights. Such an approach allows for the current findings to be considered practically as they are situated in a larger body of research. That allows some of the silos that often accompany research about sex, gender, and sexuality (see Manning, Vlasis, Dirr, Emerson, Shandy, & De Paz, 2008) to be softened so that research from different disciplines can be used together for practical application.

Families. As the data presented in this study reflect, family members should not be afraid to acknowledge a need for safe sex, but they also should not dwell on the topic. The responses of some family members discussed in this study—such as the mother who was afraid to hug her son after he came out to her—demonstrate that fear is still a possibility and education about sexual health is still in order on a large scale. Moreover, a family member exhibiting care and creating a space of openness is ideal. Even if the person receiving a disclosure feels as if their love and care for the LGB person is evident, that same vulnerable person coming out might not see things in the same light. Hearing explicit affirmation can be helpful. Family members interested in creating an open and affirming environment for those coming out to them should consider Manning's (2014) research exploring positive and negative communicative behaviors in coming out conversations (see tables 3.3 and 3.4).

Table 3.3.   Positive Communicative Behaviors in Coming Out Conversations (Manning, 2014)

Behavior	Defined	Representative Dialogue or Action
Open Communication Channels	The receiver of a coming out disclosure invites future discussion about the revealer's sexual and romantic identity	"And, so you know, any time you want to talk about this aspect of your life I am open to hearing about it!"
Affirming Direct Relational Statements	The receiver of a coming out disclosure directly and explicitly expresses value of the person and their relationship	"Mikey, I'm just happy you told me. I love you and I am so proud to be your mother!"
Laughter and Joking	The receiver of a coming out disclosure uses gentle humor to show acceptance	"Damn, Maria. You're so hot, you make me want to be a lesbian, too! Seriously, though, congrats, and thanks for telling me!"
Nonverbal Immediacy	The receiver of a coming out disclosure uses appropriate touch as a means of showing affection	Hugs, taking a hand while talking, rubbing a shoulder or arm while talking

Table 3.4. Negative Communicative Behaviors in Coming Out Conversations (Manning, 2014)

Behavior	Defined	Representative Dialogue or Action
Expressing Denial	The receiver of a coming out disclosure asks about or insists that the LGB person is confused about her or his identity	"You're not a lesbian. That new girl you're hanging out with has just convinced you that you are!"
Religious Talk	The receiver of a coming out disclosure invokes religion as a critique of identity	"It just goes against the Bible."
Inappropriate Questions, Comments, or Concerns	The receiver of a coming out disclosure asks questions, makes comments, or expresses concerns that violate privacy expectations	"So, I just need to know, how do two girls do it? It doesn't even make sense since, you know, there's nothing to stick in."
Shaming Statements	The receiver of a coming out disclosure directly admonishes judgment toward the LGB person	"Well, I'm sorry, but that gay stuff is just disgusting."
Aggression	The receiver of a coming out disclosure displays physical or verbal behaviors that are intimidating or hostile	"I'm going to kick the shit out of you, you disgusting faggot!"

As those suggestions indicate, it is not only important for the receiver of a coming out disclosure to be mindful about the situation, but the person disclosing can also take steps to better prepare him or herself for what might happen in such conversations.

Health care interaction. The findings of this study also allow considerations for health care providers. First, they should be sensitive when bringing up HIV tests or other HIV/AIDS-related topics. As the data reflect, gay and bisexual men were insulted and felt discriminated against when physicians suggested they should be tested for HIV. Physicians and other health care professionals might find themselves frustrated by the participants' interpretation of an invitation for an HIV test to be discriminatory, as the U.S. Preventitive Services Task Force recommendation statement suggests that clincians screen everyone for HIV infection, and not only men who sleep with men, who is aged fifteen to sixty-five (Moyer, 2013). As that indicates, the discrimination perceived by gay and bisexual men could very well be nonexistent—but, given that they probably do not see other patients' interaction with health care professionals, men who sleep with men might not understand that this as invitation is offered to a large body of patients that includes others beyond them. In other words, a larger distal discourse related to HIV and AIDS is coming into play with the proximal discourse between patient and doctor, and that allows gay or bisexual patients to feel as if they are being discriminated against even when they are not.

One simple fix for this problem is for health care providers to educate their patients. A statement such as, "You know, the U.S. Preventative Services Task Force recommends that we encourage just about everyone, regardless of age, gender, race, or sexual orientation, to be tested for HIV," could help to make it evident that it is not a recently disclosed sexual orientation driving that invitation but a larger standard of health care that applies to multiple people of multiple backgrounds. Additionally, health care providers should consider that even if they feel as if they are personable with patients and perhaps forging a relationship, that their identities as health care providers creates a presentational-rhetorical role (Manning, 2014) that constructs a systemic power difference where clinicians are seen as all-seeing, scientifically informed experts. Moreover, that role of health care provider almost certainly is enmeshed with professional standards, and so a tension between what a health care professional must say *professionally* versus what they need to say *personally* is likely at play. Health care providers must be cognizant of this tension and how it comes into play with the expectations and understandings of patients who often feel vulnerable in health care settings.

As this all establishes, it is not always so much about the actual coming out conversation itself—although that is quite important—but about the setting or scene created for the conversation to occur. For example, the forms that people fill out prior to seeing a health care provider often provide options for relational status that exclude same-sex relationships (Hitchcock & Wilson, 1992). Choices often include *single, married,* or even *widowed* that, at best, assume marriage equality is in play and, at worst, does not allow for the idea that nonheterosexual identities exist. Extending options could allow for affirmation prior to interaction that allows coming out as LGB to a health care provider to be more welcoming. As some participants also indicated, waiting rooms are not always a welcome space for LGB people. As Hitchcock and Wilson (1992) note, something as simple as the presence of LGB-oriented magazines (such as *The Advocate* or *Out*) can allow for a friendly environment.

As the data reflect, this welcoming environment must also lead to welcoming interaction. Almost thirty years ago Kus (1985) found that LGB people reported experiences similar to what the men in this study articulated: that many doctors seemed to behave as if they never had any interaction with other nonheterosexual people. Kus's suggestion is echoed here: the easiest way to remedy this lack of experience and to rid one's self of negative preconceptions is by talking with other LGB people. That might seem like a challenge for health care professionals who feel they have no LGB friends or family members—but making those connections can be as easy as sponsoring focus groups where LGB folk share their experiences. Another possibility is volunteering to present to LGB-oriented groups to talk about a health topic they may have an interest in hearing about, especially a topic that is not a stereotypical choice. Short of any research evidence about interacting with LGB communities, these options can present a good-faith effort to listen and learn.

Past research has indicated that those with nonheterosexual orientations might have anxieties about sharing their romantic or sexual identities with health care providers because they fear their privacy will be compromised and those who they might not be ready to or do not want to share their identity with—whether that be friends, coworkers, or community members—will react negatively (Tiemann, Kennedy, & Haga, 1998). This concern is particularly prevalent in smaller communities, especially if specialized care is being sought and provider choice is limited. Just as privacy management of sexual and romantic identity is a systemic concern, so too is the issue of sexual health. Manning (2014) argues for a holistic communicology of sexual health that is inclusive of both relational aspects of sexuality as well as medicalized and mental health concerns so that connections across all areas can be made and, consequently, both personalized and public health programs aimed at sexual health improved. The data presented in this chapter certainly lend credence to this idea, but future studies can probe even deeper into these connections. For example, research on lesbian women's health alone demonstrate that their health is correlated with increased risk for alcohol and drug problems, suicide attempts, depression, and physical or verbal abuse (Lehmann, Lehmann, & Kelly 1998). What—at the cognitive, relational, and cultural levels—is occurring to allow such statistics? New studies measuring cultural progress would be of benefit, as would studies empirically demonstrating the connections between LGB health and various cultures. Even in the face of increased civil rights and acceptance, a holistic sense of research about LGB persons and their sexual health is imperative.

A CONCLUDING THOUGHT: SEEING BEYOND THE SEXUAL

Along those lines, and in the interest of a holistic communicology of sexual health, it might be time to retire the terms *sexual orientation* or *sexual identity* and replace them with *romantic and sexual identity*. Such a turn would avoid the heteronormative trappings of otherness in language about nonheterosexual people (Foster, 2008; Manning, 2009) and allow them both romantic and sexual identities while still acknowledging that LGB people—as with people in general—can have a sexual existence without notions of romance being involved (Manning, 2011). Given the connection between discourses of coming out across contexts—especially considering that they are constitutive of all experiences as they are lived in different places and at different times—it could be helpful for all to remember that talk between health care providers and their patients might seem to be ostensibly about health, but these conversations are part of a larger series of conversations about romantic and sexual identity that LGB people experience (Adams, 2011; Manning, 2014). Perhaps that is the biggest lesson imbued by this research: A coming out conversation is never in isolation, and its impact never limited to the only the people involved. The experience is carried by the participants into future interactions, making the connections between health, individuals, relationships, and cultures inevitable and enduring.

NOTE

1. The author would like to thank Teresa Heinz Housel for her helpful feedback offering possible directions for this piece.

Shaping Self with the Doctor

The Construction of Identity for Trans Patients

Katy Ross, Juliann C. Scholl, and Gina Castle Bell

*V*isiting a doctor can be a nerve-racking experience that some individuals try to avoid altogether. The communication strategies that practitioners employ in the doctor's office play a significant part in both patients' health care decisions and their choice to return for future health care. Transgender health care is a relatively new field in which a majority of doctors seem to be unfamiliar. Because of this novelty, many doctors might be unaware of the proper terminology to use when treating a transgender patient, as well as what meaning their behaviors convey. Overall, the ways in which transgender individuals discuss their body or ailments, along with the communication doctors use concerning the patient's body or ailments, could substantially affect a transgender individual's identity.

Transgender individuals have the task of rationalizing which parts of their former identity to merge with the new identity being formed each day. According to Jackson (2002), identity is relational. This means that both personal and social identity is partially dependent upon interactions with others in society. It is reasonable to assume, then, that doctors help shape a transgender individual's health identity through the language they choose when communicating with the transgender patient.

Research has yet to make the connection between patient behavior and provider behavior as a significant source of transgender health identity development (Newfield, Hart, Dibble, & Kohler, 2006). To fill this gap in transgender literature, a pilot study consisting of five qualitative interviews was conducted with self-identifying transgender individuals who have had experience in the health communication context. The goal of this study is to significantly impact transgender literature through findings about the development of health identity for transgender individuals.

Framed through Identity Negotiation Theory (INT), this pilot study explores how transgender patients negotiate their health identity with their doctors (Ting-Toomey, 2005). The purpose of this study was to learn the ways in which doctors and transgender patients, in the health communication context, enhance and hinder the transgender patient's identity development. Particular health-related behaviors such as endorsing stereotypes or coping with experiences can potentially add to or take away from a transgender patient's health identity. This pilot study aims to distinguish these influential behaviors enacted by the transgender patient and the health professional.

LITERATURE REVIEW

Many definitions of transgender (trans) and transsexuality tend to center on the medical aspects of a patient's gender transition, such as surgery and hormone therapy. It is noteworthy that medicine factors into some trans persons' identities because it is often tied to and dependent upon the medical treatments available to them (Keller, 1999). Issues of gender identity and role socialization are part of a trans individual's daily life. These aspects become problematic when trans individuals are assigned a dysfunctional label or a predetermined medical designation different from their preferred titles (e.g., preferring to be called "she" instead of being called "he"). The desire and the need to transition to a different biological sex often are problematized through the medicalization of this process, as well as the implication that "transsexualism" is a disorder.

In the following sections, key terms will be defined to establish a mutual terminology. Then, three main areas of transgender literature will be discussed. Included in these areas are: 1) the effects of violence and discrimination will be considered as a contributor to identity construction; 2) the communication of providers will be analyzed, including general behavior and treatment of trans patients; and 3) trans patient behavior will be explored, including the areas of coping methods, gender identity, and behaviors in the doctor's office.

Establishing a Mutual Terminology: Defining Key Terms

Before beginning this larger discussion, it is vital to establish a mutual terminology from which to draw upon as transgender identity negotiation is discussed. Eight terms are defined and discussed below: Sex, gender, transgender, cisgender, gender identity, prejudice, discrimination, and transphobia. Brief examples are also provided.

First, Wood (2011) defined *sex* as "a designation based on biology" (p. 20), meaning external genitalia and internal reproductive organs. Sex is what individuals are born, male or female, and gender is how individuals learn to act or express themselves, as masculine or feminine. Second, a definition of *gender* is, "not something we have, but something that we do, over and over again in one setting or another" (Allen, 2004, p. 41). Gender is a learned behavior to express self-identification, as masculine or feminine. Third, *transgender* (trans or trans★) is used to describe those individuals "who identify psychologically or emotionally with the sex different from their biological or legally defined sex" (Allen, p. 41) and seek temporary or permanent physical changes to live as their desired sex. Trans can serve as an umbrella term encompassing transsexuals, intersex, and cross-dressers, among others. Moreover, some individuals use the term "trans★" to include all identities in the gender spectrum, such as noncisgender, gender queer, two-spirit gender, gender fluid, and many others (Killermann, 2013). *Cisgender*, according to Schilt and Westbrook (2009) is the term used to denote those individuals who are "gender normal" (p. 41), meaning that their gender identity and biological makeup match and are completely female or male. This term is slowly coming into the forefront of language used in the transgender community and by scholars who study transgender issues.

Fourth, the term *gender identity* refers to "one's sense of being a member of a particular sex" (Meyerowitz, 2002, p. 115). In other words, gender identity is how, and to what degree, an individual chooses to express masculinity or femininity.

Fifth, *prejudice* is referred to as holding empathy for or against affiliates of particular cultural groups (Castle Bell, 2012). Therefore, those that are prejudiced against members of the trans community can be said to have *trans prejudice*. Sixth, *discrimination* is defined as something that "involves committing an act or offense based on one's affinity for or against some particular cultural group" (Castle Bell, p. 7). Specifically, discrimination is acting upon the trans prejudice an individual holds, via violence or harassment. Finally, literally defined, *transphobia* is the fear of trans individuals. More specifically, transphobia is understood as "institutional, societal, and individual-level discrimination against transgender persons" (Nemoto, Bodeker, & Iwamoto, 2011, p. 1980).

Discrimination: Violence and Harassment

Discrimination can happen in a number of places, comes in many forms, can be enacted by any person, and can have many effects on the physical and mental state of a trans individual. Heath (2006) reports that harassment or violence is experienced by approximately 60 percent of transgender individuals. There are many ways in which discrimination can occur.

Places. Generally, public spaces are the prime locations for discrimination to occur. Some examples would be schools, airports, media, department stores, parking lots, online chat rooms, and restrooms (Beemyn & Rankin, 2011). Another common area where transgender individuals are the target of discriminatory behaviors is health facilities (Kenagy, 2005). There have been many testimonies given describing specific experiences with harassment and discrimination. Unfortunately, very few experiences are reported because of the fear or distrust of law enforcement (Sheridan, 2009). Many trans individuals choose to avoid police involvement altogether on discrimination experiences because of the potential physical abuse that police officers will present.

Forms. Physical violence is not the only type of discrimination present in trans individuals' lives because it also comes in other forms. A few of these can include both direct and indirect verbal slurs, sexual abuse, threats of physical violence, refusal of services, and threats to expose trans identity (Beemyn & Rankin, 2011). These issues of discrimination can be present in any of the public spaces mentioned. However, Wilkinson (2006) reports that refusal of services is common in the health realm, including denial of health insurance coverage and health care services. Because most doctors lack a general knowledge of trans-related issues, they often falsely categorize the trans patients and give irrelevant care or no care at all. Discrimination can come from any set of individuals that, knowingly or unknowingly, hold a level of transphobia.

Perpetrators. Any one person or group of people is capable of committing acts of discrimination. Identified perpetrators include children and teenagers, clinicians, strangers, police officers, colleagues and supervisors, family members, teachers and fellow students, church members, friends, and neighbors, among myriad others (Beemyn & Rankin, 2011). Discrimination is not limited to a specific type of person or a certain relationship with the trans individual. In fact, according to Beemyn and Rankin, the most frequent group of persons to cause distress through discrimination was strangers; however, following closely behind are coworkers. Regardless of the person(s) executing the form(s) of discrimination, the harmful effects still stand for trans individuals.

Effects. There are many effects of discrimination for trans individuals that can include physical aspects, such as severe beatings, rape, or murder (Sloop, 2000). Other effects could include internalized transphobia, concealment, and expectations of future violence (Testa, Sciacca, Wang, Hendricks, Goldblum, Bradford, & Bongar, 2012). Furthermore, Wilkinson (2006) notes that additional effects of discrimination for trans individuals can involve instilled fear, homelessness, suicide, self-esteem issues, or mental health disparities. Sadly, some of the worst cases exemplifying the results of discrimination end in murder, commonly with a combination of severe beatings and/or rape, like that of Brandon Teena. As described by Sloop, Brandon was a trans-man living in Nebraska and did anything he had to do to get by and continue his life as a man, unnoticed. He proceeded to steal credit cards and write fraudulent checks until he was caught and thrown in the women's jail under his given female name. Questions were raised, and when Brandon refused to reveal his former female identity, his "friends" beat, raped, and killed him. According to Wilkinson, "at least one transgendered person is murdered per month in the United States" (p. 193). Although these effects might vary, with some being extreme and others seemingly less detrimental, all impact identity.

Provider Communication

A trans individual's health identity can be hindered or enhanced by the provider-patient interaction. When communicating with trans patients in the health communication context, health providers engage in general and treatment-specific behaviors that impact trans individuals. General behaviors can be described as the interpersonal interactions with the trans patient in the office, particularly during regular visits. Included in these general behaviors are prejudice and stereotypes. Treatment behaviors are those that involve the physical care or assignment of surgical or body-altering remedies. General and treatment behaviors are reviewed in the following sections.

General Behaviors. Considering the strict gender binary society tends to promote, the stereotypes revolving around male and female, or masculine and feminine, are difficult to shed when approached by a trans individual. Providers sometimes have a tendency to bring the daily stereotypes they hold about individuals into the doctor's office. This applies especially to those belonging to the trans community. For instance, a team of health professionals working on an individual's gender transition questioned a FTM's (female-to-male) decision to transition on the basis of whether the members thought he would be attractive with the outcome (Ramsey, 1996). The personal opinions of surgeons can hinder a trans individual's positive identity development. On the contrary, using the preferred gender terminology with a trans individual, among other positive behaviors, functions to create an environment supportive of disclosure (Aramburu Alegria, 2011).

There are common stereotypes that follow the trans community as a whole, such as the belief that all trans individuals opt for full surgery, including hormone replacement therapy, top surgery (e.g., the addition or removal of breasts), and bottom surgery (e.g., alteration of the genital system). Aramburu Alegria (2011) posits that transition is constantly evolving and can be executed differently for each individual. Transition can include full surgery for some, but might not include any surgery for others. Providers should not assume all trans individuals seek the same end result. To create a more supportive environment for trans individuals, Aramburu Alegria makes three key recommendations: Ask trans individuals their preferred name, be conscious of gendered pronoun usage, and be aware of gender labeling language. The more encouraging the environment is in the doctor's office, the more likely a trans patient is to disclose more information and be less resistant with physician requests and directives.

Treatment Behaviors. Health providers' prejudice and stereotypes not only impact the general behaviors in the health communication context, but they also influence the treatment trans individuals receive to progress through transition. Transition is not a simple process; trans individuals can go through many steps to present successfully as their preferred gender. Providers hold the responsibility of fostering an empathetic atmosphere as well as supplying adequate health treatments to trans patients to make transitioning less difficult. The World Professional Association for Transgender Health's (WPATH) standards for health care to transition include: "(a) evaluation by a mental health professional; (b) hormonal therapy; and (c) year of real-life experience, or living in the desired gender for one year prior to Sexual Reassignment Surgery (SRS)" (Aramburu Alegria, 2011, p. 178). These criteria exist for a trans individual to be able to receive any type of surgery to further the transition process. Due to these WPATH standards, trans individuals depend upon health professionals to further them along through each step of their transition. Health professionals can prevent or hinder such progression. Research has shown trans individuals face many barriers to health care including embarrassment, fear of prejudice, and anxiety over being "outed" to family members (Aramburu Alegria, 2011, p. 178). Health professionals are advised to be concerned with these health barriers and how to prevent them, even the barriers they themselves present. Of special interest should be the risks resulting from each of these potentially harmful behaviors.

Trans Patient Behaviors

Doctors are not the only individuals who influence the development of trans individuals' health identities. Trans individuals themselves serve a central role in shaping their own health identity. As patients, trans individuals face unique challenges in the health communication context and have been shown to use specific interactional coping methods. In this pilot study, coping methods are specifically applied to interactions with the doctor. Gender identity is an area trans individuals must navigate in order to effectively communicate their wants and needs to doctors, and this often requires a more active role in the health communication process for the trans individual. Each of these topics is discussed in the following sections.

Coping Behaviors. Doctors' positive or negative communication toward their patients requires a response from the trans individual. When faced with a situation that requires coping, trans individuals usually need to vent in excitement or remorse, depending on the impact of their doctor's communication behavior. Immediate family and close friends are generally some of the main sources of support for trans individuals, similar to other marginalized groups, such as gays, lesbians, and bisexuals. Most people, regardless of gender identity, turn to others for support and advice when in a tough situation.

One study identified the two categories of coping methods that trans individuals use as being *avoidant* and *facilitative coping*. *Avoidant coping* consists of avoidance of emotional response, avoidance of the problem itself, avoidance of attachment to the outcome, or overeating or drinking (Budge, Adelson, & Howard, 2013). Avoidance techniques can be helpful to overcome the problems faced; however, they could potentially have long-term effects on the trans individual's self-esteem and/or identity. *Facilitative coping* transpires when the trans individual pursues social support, learns new abilities, shifts behavior to acclimate constructively, and finds different options for happiness (Budge et al.). Coping methods are useful in most situations; however, some situations might not allow trans individuals to be out in every aspect of their daily lives. This suppression of identity can be detrimental and harmful to the trans individual's psyche.

Gender Identity. Claiming a gender identity is assumed in today's society. Most individuals have no need to make extra efforts to prove their gender. However, trans individuals live in a society that largely chooses to see only two genders: male and female. Trans individuals break this mold of a binary and claim their position outside, around, and in the middle of this gender dichotomy. A trans individual's gender identity can also significantly add to how they see their health identity. For example, a trans woman who largely embraces her feminine gender identity might refer to her annual physical check-up as a "well woman exam."

Some trans individuals prefer to transition and fall back into the shadows of heteronormativity. However, there are individuals who choose to hold their trans identity, as their gender identity, with pride. Some notable examples of these individuals in the past and present are Christine Jorgenson, Kate Bornstein, and Susan Stryker. Claiming and recognizing trans identity leads to higher levels of happiness in life, including psychological freedom from fear, pressures to conform, and shame regarding suppression of identity (Bockting, Robinson, Benner, & Scheltema, 2010). Whether a trans individual identifies as man/woman or trans, accepting the trans identity can be crucial to creating a sense of self. John Money, one of the contributing scholars who helped expand the idea of gender in the 1950s, has been quoted as saying, "The process of achieving a complete gender identity is a developmental progression, beginning with genetic foundations and terminating with social learning" (Meyerowitz, 2002, p. 117). This point suggests that gender identity is a social construct. As society learns about trans issues, trans individuals learn about themselves. Gender identity is shaped and adapted in all social situations, including the doctor's office.

In the Doctor's Office. The communicative choices patients make in the medical interaction have implications for how they might convey and understand their role as a patient. Most trans patients no longer act as bystanders in the medical process but rather take on more active roles. Keller (1999) argues that the doctor-patient influence in trans-medical contexts is not a linear dialogue. Rather, trans patients who seek SRS have arguably influenced the screening process and the steps to prepare for the physical transformation. For example, a patient seeking permanent gender changes could disclose information during counseling and screening that increases the likelihood of being approved for surgery (Billings & Urban, 1982). Because of the possibility of this feedback loop between the patient and the provider, Keller questions whether trans patients are victims of medical rhetoric or active participants.

According to Dewey (2008), patients shape their behavior with the doctor according to how they perceive others view them, including the doctor. This altering of behavior can be to ensure the proper and preferred treatment is given and to prevent any pejorative classifications from taking place. Doctors are still learning about the medical treatments involved in transgenderism. Dewey states:

> Doctors' lack of knowledge regarding hormones and surgeries is a commonly held concern as many doctors are not well-versed on these issues as either medical or personal choices. Some trans individuals take the time to learn about issues related to their health so they are better prepared to discuss these topics with doctors (Dewey, p. 1352).

As some trans individuals learn more about their medical situations, they can find themselves having to educate the doctors on trans issues.

Nevertheless, a great deal of the discrimination that transgender individuals experience takes place within the medical setting (Dewey, 2008); this includes medical treatments and procedures sought since transition has taken place. In addition to stigma in everyday life, trans patients have unique hurdles with health care providers, particularly when having to prove they are an "authentic" transgender man, woman, or person. This is often the case regardless of the medical condition being addressed. Avoiding or overcoming trans victimization in the medical setting is important because the provider serves gatekeeping capacities, determining the kind and quality of treatment given, as well as making referrals to specialists.

THEORETICAL FRAMEWORK

Identity Negotiation Theory (INT) describes the countless ways in which individuals form their identity. According to Ting-Toomey (2005), INT "emphasizes that identity or reflective self-conception is viewed as the explanatory mechanism for the intercultural communication process" (p. 217). Thus, identities are shaped, reshaped, and assembled through each encounter with others. Jackson (2002) claims that identity is relational. Therefore, identity depends largely on surrounding members of society. Because gender is an everyday influence in relationships, society helps create gender identity, especially for transgender individuals (Eguchi, 2009). Health identity, then, has the potential to emerge in a doctor's office with health professionals.

Ting-Toomey (2005) introduces two types of identities that each individual maintains: personal and social identity. *Personal identity* consists of the unique characteristics an individual avows to him/herself. *Social identity* can be described as how an individual wishes others to see and treat him/her. Individuals also have a *health identity*, or tertiary identity. Tertiary identity is a variation of health identity, and is performed when an individual uses his/her illness, ailment, or health situation to help define him/herself (Harwood & Sparks, 2003). No identity stays constant; each shifts in one direction or the other based on the comments and reactions of others. People attempt to change their identities, however subtlety or drastically, according to what others say or do. Trans individuals' health identities have many influences. For instance, physicians caring for trans-specific health needs are influenced by the trans individuals' health identity.

In addition, other influences include one's self-concept, life experiences, social networks, work life, and activities that constitute one's lifestyle. These influences reflect the multiple realms of a patient's life and should not be discounted for their potential impact on one's health. For example, people who have limited social networks are likely to experience stress and anxiety when faced with life difficulties and might present physical symptoms of that stress during a doctor visit. Therefore, a person's health is dependent upon physical, social, and mental wellbeing (World Health Organization, 2004).

This definition of health assumes a biopsychosocial approach to health care. Unlike the biomedical model, which posits that ill health is a phenomenon primarily evidenced by physical causes (e.g., germs, blunt trauma), du Pré (2010) points out that the biopsychosocial model presumes that one's health is shaped by a number of physical (e.g., disease immunity, genetics), emotional (e.g., self-esteem, stress levels), and social (e.g., family issues, relationships) factors. This health care model is relevant to trans identity and health in that the medical choices patients make are significantly influenced by the social factors in their lives, which include relationships with medical professionals. The interactions trans patients have with their doctors not only influence their immediate health choices and behaviors but will also impact how they see themselves as health care seekers, and more importantly, as transgendered patients who must find a way to navigate the health care system.

RATIONALE

The goal of this study is to uncover how patient-provider interactions contribute to trans patients' development of their health identity, by supplying both positive and negative affirmations. This study seeks to reveal the ways in which trans patients negotiate their health identity in the doctor's office. In addition, given the reported discrimination and mistreatment that many trans patients receive from their providers, it is this study's intent to discover common patterns or potential themes of such behaviors on the part of providers. Such insights will help providers and educators improve their communication with trans patients and other vulnerable individuals. Therefore, we pose the two research questions:

> **RQ1:** How do trans patients negotiate their health identities with their doctors?

> **RQ2:** What forms of discrimination do trans individuals report experiencing when communicating with providers?

METHODOLOGY

Participants

The participants in this study included those who self-identity as transgender and have taken either temporary or permanent steps to present as the desired gender. These individuals came from various locations around the United

States. Five self-identifying transgender individuals were interviewed. The age range of participants was twenty-two to thirty-one years old. All participants fell along a continuum of positions in transition. This means that some individuals were further in transition with potential for a completed SRS, whereas others had just started hormone replacement therapy. Of our five participants, two had been on hormone replacement therapy for under one year and three for between two and five years. Only two of our participants, both female-to-males, had top surgery. Two participants were seeking top surgery in the future. Only one participant expressed a direct desire to seek bottom surgery.

One of the goals of qualitative analysis is to provide a thick description or a valid account of the communicative context (Hammersley, 2008). Although we interviewed only five participants in this pilot study, interviews are considered to be valid interpretations and explanations of interpretive social science (Castle Bell, 2012). Specifically, interviews "provide accounts about the issues being studied" (Denzin & Lincoln, 2011, p. 418) and reveal important information about what the people of interest experience in certain settings (Lindlof & Taylor, 2011). Further, "qualitative research seeks depth rather than breadth. Instead of drawing from large, representative samples of an entire population, qualitative researchers seek to acquire in-depth, intimate information about a smaller group of persons" (Ambert, Adler, Adler, & Detzner, 1995, p. 880). The information gleaned from our five in-depth interviews produced rich, thick description regarding trans patients' experiences with doctors and health professionals. By thick descriptions we mean identifying the behaviors observed and the meanings attached to those behaviors by the situations and contexts in which they occur (Christians & Carey, 1989). Furthermore, sample size is less important than the "unique character of a particular situation" (Hammersley, p. 62). Finally, considering our interviews with five trans individuals, not only were we able to "produce accounts of the social world focused on particular cases" but we also "provided more general insight" into the trans-doctor-patient communication process (Hammersley, p. 62). Although we interviewed only five participants, we were able to satisfy the goals of interpretive social science.

Recruiting Participants. We used a convenience snowball sample for recruiting transgender individuals to discuss their experience in the health communication context. Convenience sampling involves using participants that the researchers find most convenient and readily available to participate in the study (Keyton, 2005). Snowball sampling "yields a study sample through referrals made among people who share or who know of others who possess some characteristic that are of research interest" (Lindlof & Taylor, 2002, p. 124). Moreover, snowball sampling is useful for interviewing individuals about a sensitive subject (Patton, 2002). The researchers accessed the individuals they knew first, and then asked for referrals from these individuals. Once the potential participants contacted the research team, they received a recruitment letter via email explaining the research and its significance.

Data Collection Methods

Developing Rapport. Due to the sensitive nature of this topic, rapport is vital for providing participants a space in which they can share openly and comfortably despite their vulnerable status. At the start of the interview, the researchers greeted and thanked the participant and reminded the participant about the information sheet they were emailed earlier, which explains the study's purpose. Thereafter, the researcher shared what participants could expect throughout the interview. Interviewees were reminded that questions would be asked about trans patient-doctor interactions. Next, the researcher shared that some questions might be sensitive and uncomfortable, but that honest thoughts about experiences were sought and valued. The participants received assurance that any question could be skipped or left unanswered, and that there was no obligation to answer any specific question. Finally, throughout the interview, the researcher maintained rapport by displaying positive, encouraging nonverbal communication cues, such as affirmative verbal fillers (e.g., "uh huh") and other feedback cues intended to show interest and appreciation.

Interviews. Interviews were this study's primary data collection method. Interviews are helpful for yielding knowledge and comprehension about the research questions under investigation from the participants' perspectives (Maxwell, 2013). Moreover, interviews enable participants to play a vital role in the data collection process by inviting them "to share their stories, examine their lived experiences, and discover information in such a way that makes participants co-researchers in creating meaning" (Castle Bell, 2012, pp. 53–54). Interviews carve space for conversation around such a sensitive topic (Silverman, 2013). In this sense, this pilot study was interested in trans individuals' lived experiences with doctors in a health communication context.

Interviews occurred via Skype or FaceTime, or over the phone. The researchers used a semistructured, or open-ended, interview schedule of primary questions that allowed for additional follow-up questions, which might not have been anticipated by the researchers (Patton, 2002). The interviews lasted approximately thirty to sixty minutes. Once rapport had been built and the interview's purpose reviewed, the researcher proceeded with the interview using a guide containing the interview questions. The researcher used a hand-held digital recording device to record the interview. The primary questions covered such issues as direct experiences with health professionals during the early and later parts of transition. At the conclusion of the interviews' question portion, the participants were given an opportunity to add any extra information and clarify all confusions. All identifying information, such as the interview digital recordings, signed inform consent forms, and typed transcripts of all interviews were stored in a password-protected computer to which only the researchers had access.

Instruments. Each interview started with a series of demographic questions asking about age, race, and highest level of education, among others. These demographic factors can potentially contribute to the data and help explain some of our findings. Demographic variables are used as controls in a study, versus primary variables, to moderate the central factors (Creswell, 2009). Using demographic questions can potentially add insights into what certain individuals said or why they were said.

Once the demographic questions were completed, the interview moved forward with the study questions. Two main sections were discussed in each interview: a) transition to transgender and b) experiences with health care as a transgender person. First, the participants were asked general questions about their transgender status. For instance, "When, and how, did you know that you were transgender?" and "What types of reactions have you encountered when disclosing your gender identity?" These types of questions contributed to creating a base layer of understanding for the researcher in each interview (see appendix A for full list of demographic and interview questions). It is important for the researcher to establish a time line of transition for each transgender individual because each individual can fall along a different point on the continuum of transition.

Second, questions were asked about the participant's experiences with health professionals during the early and later parts of transition. The researchers wanted to know about experiences prior to transition to gauge doctors' behaviors toward a cisgender individual. Sometimes individuals experience harassment or discrimination even as a child, teenager, or young adult in the health context. Questions were asked about what an ideal doctor would look like or how he or she would behave, differences in behavior of the doctor and the patient themselves, as well as how the doctors communicate with the participant. These types of questions were helpful in answering our first research question.

Methods of Data Analysis

A thematic analysis was conducted once the interviews had been fully transcribed. The goal was to find common themes apparent in each interview that demonstrated the interconnected thoughts reflected by the study (Creswell,

2009). The coding process involved reading through each interview carefully several times to locate the data's underlying meaning. The analysis followed Owen's (1984) thematic analysis using repetition, recurrence, and forcefulness to identify the categories relevant to the study. *Repetition* refers to "the duplication of key words and phrases" (Keyton, 2005, p. 41). *Recurrence* involves observing two reports that have the same thread of meaning (Keyton). Recurring thoughts or phrases do not necessarily contain identical words, but reflect the same idea of denotation. Finally, *forcefulness,* refers to being "attentive to vocal inflections and dramatic pauses that stress or subordinate some utterances" (Keyton, p. 41) during communication. Forcefulness occurs when "participants vocally emphasize certain words and phrases" (Castle Bell, 2012, p. 58). After the transcriptions were analyzed, an interpretation of the larger meaning surrounding the data was revealed (Creswell).

To assess consistency in coding, each researcher coded one or two transcripts independently. Subsequently, the researchers compared their resulting codebooks to discuss the emergent categories and resolve any differences. Coding continued with the remaining transcripts until saturation was reached. Saturation occurs when new categories and themes cease to emerge, and there are mainly repetitions and redundancies in the themes that do appear (Strauss & Corbin, 1990).

RESULTS

Identity is defined as the reflective self-conception or self-image that we each derive from our family, gender, gender identity, sexual orientation identity, social class identity, age identity, disability identity, or professional identity (Ting-Toomey, 2005). Moreover, Ting-Toomey's theory explains that individuals have basic motivational needs for identity security, identity inclusion, identity connection, and identity consistency. Finally, satisfactory identity negotiation arguably includes the feelings of being understood, respected, and affirmatively valued—all valuable outcomes, which are impacted by the ways in which patients and providers communicate (Brown, Stewart, & Ryan, 2003). There are two types of identity, personal and social identity, which together impact an individual's overall identity.

Personal identity refers to individuals' perceptions and views of themselves, the identity they claim, and overall attributes they associate with their individuated self. Therefore, having a healthy personal identity involves the ability to claim, or avow, one's own identity (Hopson, 2011). Hopson also explains that avowing one's identity empowers people to decide who they are and how they self-identify; it enables people to name themselves, to establish their own personal identity. As a result, avowal provides identity security, identity connection, and identity consistency. *Social identity* is constructed in communication with cultural and ethnic group members and includes age, class, race, region, occupation, sexual orientation, and gender identities. Here, social identity is impacted by doctor-patient communication. Maintaining a healthy social identity in the doctor's office involves communication from doctors that confers feelings of being understood, respected, and affirmatively valued.

In this study, we position individuals as cultural beings who bring their personal identities, social identities, and cultural experiences into the doctor's office (Hopson, 2011). The sum total of one's identity must also include their health identity. *Health identity* refers to the overall sense of self in terms of the physical, mental, and emotional, and it also includes one's personal and social identities. We conceptualize identity within these three realms (health, personal, and social), which together consitute the trans identity biopsychosocial health model (see figure 4.1). In this model, these three identities are

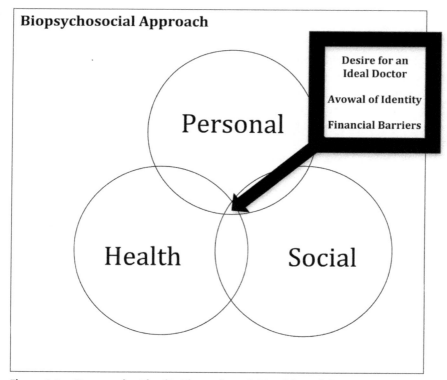

Figure 4.1.   Transgender Identity Biopsychosocial Health Model
Source: du Pré, 2010.

combined and placed under the umbrella termed "biopsychosocial model." Positioned in the middle of the model are this study's themes. This medial approach considers the needs of the whole patient, rather than simply treating the physical ailments, which can be affected by one's personal (e.g., self-esteem, individual habits or choices) and social realms (e.g., cultural group, relational status) in life.

TRANSGENDER IDENTITY BIOPSYCHOSOCIAL HEALTH MODEL

Data analysis produced the following three main themes: a) desire for an ideal doctor; b) avowal of identity; and finally, c) financial barriers as threats to identity avowal. In the following results section, themes and subthemes are presented, examples from data are provided, and all themes and subthemes are defined.

Desire for an Ideal Doctor

All participants mentioned their desire for "an ideal doctor." This conversation emerged when researchers asked how participants perceived their current doctor and the extent to which this perception matched their conception of their ideal. There are four subthemes that illustrate aspects of an ideal doctor: a) treat the whole person; b) possess ideal attributes; c) engage in identity affirmation; and finally, d) do not disconfirm trans identity by dehumanizing trans patients. Below, these subthemes are defined and examples of data illustrating their existence are presented.

Treat the Whole Person. The theme, treat the whole person, is defined within a broader health context, called the *biopsychosocial approach,* which emphasizes treating the "whole" person, rather than the person's body parts or that person's observable physical symptoms. To this end, the biopsychosocial approach takes into consideration various factors of a person's life (physical, environmental, emotional, spiritual, and social) that contribute positively and negatively to his or her health. Rather than treat the patient as little more than the disease or symptoms, a biopsychosocial attitude increases the likelihood that the patient will be treated as a whole, multifaceted person. Brandon, a thirty-one–year-old FTM identifying as Caucasian/Jewish and living in Florida, offers some statements that suggest the importance of a patient-centered, whole-patient perspective:

It is important for doctors to be knowledgeable of the trans body, um, so I don't feel, I don't know, so people feel comfortable. At lot of people are afraid to go to the hospital because they don't think they are going to get proper treatment. So it is important to be comfortable in that setting, going to a doctor, going to the hospital, so that you know they know what they are doing to take care of you.

This sense of caretaking also extends to the person as a whole, someone who possesses thoughts, experiences, and relationships in addition to the physical health concerns. Alan, a twenty-six–year-old white FTM who resides in Greenville, North Carolina, appears to support this notion when he expresses a desire for providers who are:

. . . consistent with keeping my health identity as a joint being, instead of just me being a man. Because my health revolves around so much more. Um, all of my health revolves around so much more than just, um, being a man. Because of the physical and the mental, emotional past, and all those things.

This whole person is reflected by an identity that shapes and is shaped by one's interactions with other individuals, including health care providers. A doctor who takes the biopsychosocial approach will more likely engage in communication that is confirming to a patient's health, personal, and social identities.

Ideal Attributes. In addition to ideal doctors treating the whole patient, participants explain that ideal doctors also have certain attributes. This ideal attributes theme refers to the personality and communicative qualities trans patients desire their doctors to possess. The following two examples illustrate the types of ideal attributes trans patients want in their ideal doctor. First, Thomas, a thirty-one-year-old FTM residing in San Francisco, California, expressed:

Ideally I'd like to have a supportive doctor, um. I, I'm, hmm . . . I think that as we've built our relationship together as a patient and care-provider, that I've seen her be really open to what I have to say. She's willing to engage in dialogue about, not only concerns, but research or anything, so yeah. . . . My doctor is on top of it, I would say, yeah. She knows a lot of stuff so she's a great resource, if anything. It's awesome . . . I'd really like a well-informed advocate of sorts. You know, like I do my part to stay informed as well so, I, I want them, to know, um, newest research or possibility for (transition) treatments. And then to, yeah I don't know, just to have my best interest in mind and make sure that I'm, my blood work is staying healthy, everything like that.

Here, Thomas explains his desire for an ideal doctor who engages in the following types of patient-centered communicative practices: perceived as supportive, open, willing to engage in dialogue, has patient's best interest in mind, is a great resource, and who is also a well-informed advocate regarding the transition process. In the next example of ideal attributes, Nick, a twenty-six-year-old FTM residing in Concord, North Carolina, who unlike Thomas does not have the ideal doctor, adds to Thomas' list of ideal attributes by sharing a bad experience with his current doctor:

> Uh, I'd like a doctor who would take more than twenty minutes with me . . . someone who asks me how I feel, who can say, 'OK, well, you probably have a headache because of this' and give me information. I feel like they just look at me, ask me how I am, and they give me an overall write-up instead of saying, maybe it could be this, that, I don't know. . . . You know, (I need) overall information. . . . Just the fact that I only see my doctor for ten minutes. The first time I spoke to him he gave me a prescription for testosterone. I was just like, are you going to teach me how to do it? When I asked, he said to 'just put it in a needle.' And I said, 'What type of needle?' 'You just put it in any needle, you put it in your leg, and wiggle it around.' And I'm like, . . . OK, so what type [emphasis] of needle? I was completely out of my element . . . I mean, how am I supposed to inject the needle in my body? I don't know how to do it.

Nick echoes the sentiments of other patients everywhere, as he desires more time with his doctor. Adding to time, Nick also wants his doctor to explain transition-related procedures to him, rather than merely giving him a piece of paper with instructions. He wants his doctor to embody a more hands-on approach that shows him how to do something (e.g., how to self-administer a testosterone injection), instead of simply telling him to read about it in a manual. Combined with Thomas's list of personality attributes, together these participants provide a list of supportive communicative practices that might enhance the trans-patient-doctor relationship.

Engage in Identity Affirmation. In addition to having several ideal communicative attributes, participants also explained that ideal doctors engage in identity affirmation. This subtheme emerged naturally as the trans participants discussed communication with their doctors. As our five participants spoke about their experiences with doctors, all five mentioned the "type" of doctor they would like to have. Participants explained that communication with their ideal doctor is most affirming when he or she supports their transgender identity. There are three ways in which participants expressed how ideal doctors can engage in identity affirmation: a) affirm patients as having a trans identity; b) express a desire to know more; and finally, c) communicating indifference about patients' trans status.

Affirm Patients as Having a Trans Identity. This theme is defined as providing esteem support for trans patients so they can have a sense of pride in themselves and their trans identity when they leave the doctor's office. Brandon (FTM), when asked about the impact his doctor's support had on his life, explained, "her support . . . validates it (transgender identity) I guess. I go in there and I just feel like a normal guy." In the following example, Thomas (FTM) also explains how his doctor affirmed his trans identity. However, Thomas' circumstance is unique. His doctor helped him feel comfortable identifying as transgender at each stage of transition:

> I would say that it's (going to the doctor) helped me to feel more solid in my identity. Its not just like just coming out as being transgender, like eh . . . I know that, it's totally fine to be, to identify as transgender, and not seek hormone replacement therapy . . . It just helped me feel more solid and secure in myself. It just makes me feel that I'm making the right steps forward, for me.

Thomas's doctor helped him avow his personal identity and made sure he knew that whatever transition steps he chose, any and all of them would suffice. His doctor helped him realize that transgender does not have one image after which to model. This is important because transgender individuals often occupy different stages in the transition process. Thomas's doctor provides a model for other doctors. Whether a trans patient is early in the transition process or if he or she decides not to undergo certain parts of transition, supporting a patient's trans identity is an affirmation tactic doctors can use to help trans patients avow their identity during all stages of transition.

Express Desire to Know More. In addition to engaging in communication that affirms patients' transgender identity by positioning it as normal and supporting trans patients at all transition stages, doctors can affirm trans identity in other valuable communicative ways. Specifically, participants explained that ideal doctors affirm trans identity when they *express a desire to know more about being transgender* or discussed *medically researching* the trans body. Alan (FTM) expressed how doctors could communicatively affirm trans identity best:

> And while they (doctors) were comfortable working with me, they were like, I gotta do some research first, you know. And they were very upfront and honest about that. And they would, they would ask the questions . . . And I was so thankful for that because they didn't know anything (about being transgender) and most people don't. Um, and it's not because they choose not to, it's because there's nothing out there. They were more excited and question-oriented throughout the (transition) process, um. They became more inquisitive as the (transition) process went on and (they were) more relaxed and comfortable with me and (continued) asking me questions as the process went on.

Here, Alan expresses the identity support he felt as his doctors conveyed interest in his transition process. Essentially, asking questions and expressing a desire to do research communicatively affirmed his personal identity. Given his trans status, Alan needs supportive doctors who know how to better medically treat him.

   Communication of Indifference. In addition to engaging in communication that affirms patients' transgender identity by positioning it as normal, supporting trans patients at all transition stages, and by expressing a desire to know more, doctors may be able to affirm trans identity by employing *indifference as a response*. The theme, communication of indifference, is positioned as a positive communication tactic. We conceptualize indifference as a nonchalant, uninhibited communicative response to learning a patient is transgender or wants to transition. Most people experience gender indifference, as we define it, from their doctors; other than at birth, doctors do not exclaim, "You are a wo/man, how fantastic!" Thus, nonchalantly responding to learning about transgender identity or a patient's desire to transition likely normalizes the doctor-patient-interaction for trans patients. Indifference toward one's gender identity, when it has a positive valence, normalizes rather than glorifies or ostracizes.

   Unlike the examples above, which talk about how ideal doctors affirm trans identity, Rose, a twenty-two-year-old MTF (male-to-female) residing in Fort Worth, Texas, discussed how her friends used indifference as a response to engage in identity affirmation. In the following example, Rose explains her friends' reactions to her transition decision and highlights how indifference as a response can be positive and identity affirming:

> I would say, uh, they (friends) were either support(ive) or it was indifference I received. At least in terms of discussing it (transition) as a thing that was going to happen, or existing as a thing that was going to happen, um, all of my friends . . . were pretty down with it. They didn't really mind or weren't really upset. (They voiced) Like, well, if that's what you need to do, that's what you need to do. So, in terms of peer support, I have pretty decent help, or like, uh, you know, not pure hatred and . . . it is mostly a positive thing. Um, mostly just pure acceptance.

Above, Rose explains that using indifference as a response is a communication strategy that affirmed her overall identity. Rose's discussion of indifference as an identity support tool has implications for ideal doctors and medical professionals. Perhaps ideal doctors can engage in identity affirmation by responding with indifference upon learning their patient is transgender or learning their patient desires to go through the transition process.

   This finding is extremely valuable. Although Rose's comments do not directly occur with a health professional, indifference as response can be immediately implemented by health professionals caring for trans patients. Should Rose's experience with indifference be common among the transgender community in the health context, this type of communication might enhance the trans-patient-doctor relationship. We included this example to illustrate how awareness of a particular communication strategy, indifference as response, might also immediately benefit trans-patient-doctor-communication. As such, positively valenced indifference is a transferable strategy, worthy of immediate consideration by medical and health professionals.

Avowal of Identity

In additional to treating the whole patient and desiring an ideal doctor, this second main theme highlights participants' stories that conveyed the ways in which they claim their transgender identity. Identity is defined as the reflective self-conception or self-image that we each derive from our family, gender, gender identity, sexual orientation identity, social class identity, age identity, disability identity, or professional identity (Ting-Toomey, 2005). Moreover, identity negotiation theory explains that individuals have basic motivation needs for identity security, identity inclusion, identity connection, and identity consistency. Thus, for trans patients in the doctor's office, part of having a healthy personal identity involves the ability to claim, or avow, and perform one's own identity (Hopson, 2011). Avowing one's identity provides identity security, identity connection, and identity consistency. The following three examples illustrate participants' identity avowal process.

In the first example, Rose (MTF) explains her identity avowal process by sharing how she knew she identified as transgender:

> Um . . . when I was sixteen, um, I mean, there have been kind of hints before (that age), really blatant ones . . . but the first time I was able to, like, attach a word and like, a more direct definition . . . it would probably be around sixteen. I happened to meet someone else who was trans and I was like, oh. That's the thing (I am).

For Rose, being able to pinpoint the term to describe how she was feeling helped her to avow her identity as a transgender individual. Next, like Rose, Brandon (FTM) also described the process by which he affirms his personal identity:

> Um, I knew, I've known my whole entire life that I was different. Um, but really I didn't know what it was. I didn't actually know that being transgendered existed until about 2008, um, and then it was kinda really honest with myself and I realized that how I saw myself did not fit with how I felt, so I started researching transition shortly after that.

In this final example, unlike Rose and Brent, Alan (FTM) explains how he securely claims his transgender identity as male, even though his medical identity is physically female:

> It is really hard to see yourself and identify as one thing and other people see another, um. My health identity doesn't really do my personal identity. You know, I see myself as a man; I have for years and years. But I know that my health identity will always be that of a physical female aspect . . . my gender (identity) is separate from my sex, um. I don't see that . . . as far as work—everything, I'm a man.

Illustrating the main theme of avowal of identity, Rose, Brent, and Alan expressed feeling like they were finally themselves after being able to apply the word "transgender" to their life experience. Thus in identity terms, participants' personal identities were more complete, secure, and consistent after avowing a personal, transgender identity. This kind of identity development could partially result from a more biopsychosocial, patient-centered approach that considers the impact of the patient-doctor interaction on how a trans person feels about being transgender. Additionally, this approach acknowledges the intersection of one's health with social networks, individual life choices, and close personal relationships.

Ultimately, a medical interaction that shows consideration of patients' other aspects of life contributes to their mental and emotional health, which can further affirm their trans identity. For example, asking about a trans patient's supportive social networks can help a doctor ensure that the patient is avoiding undue stress and bullying, which could lead to more physical symptoms associated with stress. In general, the ability to be secure in their transgender identity and to express it openly contributes to trans patients' overall health and wellbeing.

Financial Barriers: Threats to Identity Avowal

This main theme, financial barriers as threats to identity avowal, demonstrates the fears about transition expressed by the trans participants in this pilot study. "Financial barriers" specifically refers to not having the financial means to afford the medical treatments that are part of the transition process (e.g., hormones, surgery). Participants' narratives revealed the ways in which financial barriers function as a threat to identity avowal. Specifically, financial barriers threaten trans identity avowal because the data illustrate they impeded avowal and potentially slow the transition process. The biopsychosocial approach is relevant here in that the financial inability to proceed through gender transition can have implications for how trans individuals are perceived and treated by their social networks as their preferred gender. Such implications can also exist within the personal realm, as in one's choice of clothing or activities that are perceived to reflect one's gender identity. Discussion of threats to identity avowal emerged naturally in the data collection process when researchers asked participants what if anything, hindered their transition process.

In the following example, Rose (MTF) described the ways in which finances hindered her transition process:

> Basically, finances were a huge stumbling block . . . [I am] about twenty-eight months [into transition], something like that. Um, and that's all I can really afford to do now, in the position of finances. The other kind of big (transition) step for me, uh, would be bottom surgery . . . um, but it looks like those are probably going to be years off at this point, you know, due to finances.

Rose explains not having the finances necessary for further transition surgeries she wants. Identity negotiation theory (INT) provides a context regarding why financial barriers might threaten personal identity or the ability to avow one's trans identity. The threat inherent in not being able to transition fully is represented in assumption two of INT, which emphasizes a person's basic identity need for identity consistency, identity security, and identity inclusion (Ting-Toomey, 2005). The inability to financially support transition might impact some trans individuals' overall ability to securely avow their identity.

Thus, lack of finances can be perceived as a threat to identity, which might cause individuals to experience emotional insecurity or vulnerability in terms of identity avowal. Trans individuals are cultural beings who bring their values, beliefs, norms, practices, and personal experiences with them into the doctor's office (Hopson, 2011). It is possible that these feelings of identity held by trans patients will transfer to the doctor visit.

DISCUSSION

The purpose of this study was to determine how a trans individual's identity is negotiated in the doctor's office through the use of affirmative practices or disconfirming behaviors. We found significant data describing the ideal doctor for a trans patient, including the ideal attributes of the doctor, the ways in which a trans individual's identity is avowed, and the financial barriers to completing transition. The model, which positions the three types of identities (personal, social, and health) within a biopsychosocial context, addresses the first research question: How do trans patients negotiate their health identities with their doctors? The second research question asks what forms of discrimination trans individuals report when communicating with providers. The three main themes address financial barriers and disconfirmation, as well as affirmative behaviors that help to reduce discrimination. Although these results are important and helped to answer our research questions, this study has some limitations. Below, we explain the limitations, implications for research, and offer a few applied implications and recommendations for professionals who are likely to interact with trans individuals.

Limitations

First, it could be argued that the number of participants we were able to interview is relatively low, even for this study's emic approach. However, given the stigmatization many trans people experience in their everyday lives, the number of people willing to speak to us should not be considered unusual, especially because the individuals interviewed were strangers to us, having been referred to us by personal and professional contacts. Ultimately, transcriptions from the five interviewees yielded greater understanding of participants' "experience, knowledge, and worldviews" (Lindlof & Taylor, 2011, p. 173) and provided an invaluable baseline for future researchers to further explore this population. Ultimately, the five interviews are valuable forms of qualitative inquiry because they increase knowledge about the ways in which trans individuals communicate with health professionals. In all, the amount of data gathered was disproportionately large given the number of people who were interviewed.

Another potential limitation was the inability to interview the participants face-to-face. Instead, all interviews were conducted over video chat, like Skype or FaceTime, or over the phone, and they were all audio-recorded. These computer-mediated interview settings were necessary because it was difficult to recruit interviewees in northwest Texas, a region which tends to be conservative and sometimes hostile toward individuals who identify as trans, trans★, or LGBTQ. Moreover, Lindlof and Taylor (2011) explain that computer-mediated and phone interviews are equally valuable as face-to-face interviews because they allow researchers to interview participants in real-time. Further, Lindlof and Taylor clarify that phone interviews, which we position as similar to Skype and FaceTime for the same reason, "may help the participant feel freer to disclose personal information, because they don't expect to meet the researcher again" (p. 190).

To make the telephone/video interviews as media-rich as possible, we used paralinguistic and other verbal and nonverbal behaviors that are typically associated with immediacy, tolerance, and genuine interest (e.g., paraphrasing, vocal fillers, affirming responses such as "I see" and "Uh huh"). Most interviewees thanked us for how we handled the interviews, which strongly suggests that the telephone/video chats were not a significant barrier to the interpersonal connections we likely made with the participants.

The study might also be limited in the lack of questions we asked about finances and financial barriers faced by trans people. Sanchez, Sanchez, and Danoff (2009) point out that money is often a limiting factor for many people when seeking health care, and the lack of it is a commonly reported barrier for trans patients. In our study, for example, Rose disclosed that she wanted to start her hormone therapy at age eighteen but had to delay treatments because she could not yet afford them. That the topic of finances was not included in our interview protocol could have caused us to overlook additional financial barriers that would have otherwise been reported.

Theoretical Implications

This study yields three significant implications to theory, specifically INT: a) the Trans Identity Biopsychosocial Model created through this study helps to extend INT; b) INT serves as a framework to treat trans health as a whole; and c) trans individuals can benefit in three main ways by grasping the concept of INT.

First, INT is extended through the use of the Trans Identity Biopsychosocial Model. This model takes a holistic approach to identity within the trans community. It considers the two primary identities in INT, social and personal, and adds health identity to create an all-inclusive interpretation of identity. According to our model, as cultural beings, individuals bring their understanding of their personal and social identity, as well as their cultural experiences, into the doctor's office. This concept can be applied to any topic surrounding identity; therefore, other themes could connect the three identities to establish a biopsychosocial viewpoint of identity in any given setting.

Second, INT, as it is used in this study, is a suitable framework that health care professionals can use to treat their trans patients and view identity as a crucial part to health care. When identity is disconfirmed, physical, mental, and social health can decline. Individuals seek to be understood, respected, and valued in any setting, but more importantly, in the doctor's office (Ting-Toomey, 2005). For instance, when a trans individual goes in to see the doctor, simply being called by the preferred pronouns can significantly increase that individual's wellbeing. When health care professionals recognize that they play a role in the negotiation and formation of identity for trans individuals, treatment satisfaction is likely to increase.

Finally, a blanket understanding of INT can aid trans individuals in three ways: a) they can better communicate their needs with health care professionals; b) they can understand themselves better; and c) they can learn to relate better to society at large. First, trans individuals can learn to communicate their needs to their doctors if they have a fuller understanding of how identity contributes to health care. For instance, if a trans individual's social identity has been scarred and they recognize that, they will be able to communicate that to their doctor in order to improve overall health. Second, trans individuals can gain a better understanding of themselves through INT. Having a better sense of self has an intrinsic value. Trans individuals have the potential to feel more solid and confident in their identity as a person and as a trans individual through the concepts presented in INT. Finally, by understanding the self better through INT, a trans individual is likely able to communicate easier with the larger portion of society. Recognizing the social and personal identity as it changes can improve everyday interactions with others.

Research Implications

The findings from our study present specific research implications, one of which is the value and utility of qualitative interviews with trans people who seek health care. The transition processes and experiences of trans individuals are still misunderstood by some members of the medical community. Personal interviews can continue to provide insights into trans patients' biopsychosocial needs, especially when studied in tandem with more quantitative measures, such as quality of life (Newfield et al., 2006). Such richer findings are not only for the providers' benefit and use, but they also can contribute to the literature on transgender health care. Additionally, Newfield et al. also encourage the use of interviews on a longitudinal scale to capture more complete histories of individuals going through the gender-transition process.

Second, as future studies investigate health identity among trans individuals, as well as further explore the role of identity negotiation in gender transition, researchers could refine further themes such as ours into observable and measurable variables for more quantitative investigations. For instance, causal or correlational relationships might be explored between the impact of financial barriers and avowal of trans identity, which could have practical implications regarding access to transition-related health care. In addition, such variables can be linked with measures of quality of life and trans patient satisfaction (Bockting et al., 2010), as well as other demographic markers, such as ethnicity, age, and socioeconomic status, which might further impact patient access to and quality of care.

Research also needs to continue to investigate the prevalence of HIV/ AIDS among transgender populations, as well as factors associated with infection, such as social isolation, economic marginalization, and misperceptions of HIV/AIDS risk (Herbst, Jacobs, Finlayson, McKleroy, Neumann, & Crepaz, 2008). Because health identity arguably reflects and affects health care decisions and everyday choices, more focused investigations of risk factors associated with HIV/AIDS and other infections are needed. Studies that acknowledge the intersection of health, social, and personal identities can enable researchers to discover and test more effective ways to administer to patients' emotional needs, educate patients on risk factors and treatment options, and identify segmented at-risk populations in the transgender community.

Applied Implications and Recommendations to Educators and Health Care Professionals

Based on our study's findings, we make concrete recommendations for enhancing the experience of trans patients, reducing stigma associated with transgender identity, and educating both trans patients and providers on positive health outcomes. First is to make more available and prevalent curricular programs and seminars that educate providers on trans patients' medical needs. Such programs should include explanations and definitions of transgender terms (e.g., cisgender, MTF, FTM, gender queer); discussions of gender-conscious and inclusive language recommended for health care environments; physiological considerations and common treatments (hormone therapy, top surgery, bottom surgery); interacting with trans patients on nontransition medical issues; trans issues unique to children, adolescents, and older adults; mental health and psychiatric needs; health disparities experienced by trans patients; and spiritual and religious considerations. Such programs should not be available only to physicians and nursing staff but also to any health care personnel (e.g., insurance and claims specialists, receptionists, custodial staff) who have contact with trans patients. Medical schools, hospitals, student wellness centers, and other entities might find ways to create incentives for attending such programs.

In addition to obtaining more education, health practitioners can do things to make their offices and facilities more trans-friendly and inclusive. Policies regarding communication with LGBTQ patients can be included in employee handbooks. For instance, office personnel should be encouraged to call patients by their preferred names, which might be different than what is listed on their medical records and legal documents. Personnel can also be coached to use "partner" or "significant other" instead of talking about a patient's "husband" or "wife." In general, patients should be allowed to stipulate how they want to be addressed or what to be called. Such policies can be considered as equally important as those regarding patient privacy.

Physical changes can also be made within the medical setting, such as intake and admissions forms that include more inclusive gender categorizations.

Ard and Makadon (2013), writing for the Fenway Institute, recommend three questions for gathering gender-related information on forms:

1. What is your current gender identity? (check all that apply) __male __female __transgender male/trans man/FTM __transgender female/ trans woman/MTF __genderqueer __additional category (please specify) __decline to answer
2. What sex were you assigned at birth? (check one) __male __female __decline to answer
3. What pronouns do you prefer (e.g., he/him, she/her)? _____

Making gender-neutral restrooms available is another step toward creating a more inclusive medical office. Instead of building an additional restroom or reconstructing the office space, gender-neutral restroom designations can be used to replace the common male/female signs.

We also make recommendations for trans patients. We strongly advocate that patients be prepared to educate their providers or explain terms, jargon, and experiences that might be unique to trans individuals and unfamiliar to doctors. For example, not all doctors, and even those who see trans patients regularly, know what *trans★* means, which could create confusion if the patient were to write this term on an intake or admission form. In addition to explaining terms, trans patients should not hesitate to alert their providers to side effects of certain treatments; such alerts could help their doctors watch for similar conditions in other trans patients. By trans patients taking the initiative to be prepared to educate their doctors, they are taking part in the expansion of knowledge in health care and the general population alike.

The biopsychosocial approach assumes, among other things, that patients can be active participants in their health care and medical interactions. Although patients vary in the level or amount of partnership they seek, they can learn ways to express their desire for more input in their health care decisions. For instance, when being prescribed hormone therapy, patients can ask for all options in how that therapy is administered (e.g., pills, gels, injections) and ask for the advantages and disadvantages of each option. Patients can also adopt the "Ask Me 3" model (National Patient Safety Foundation, 2013), which is designed to equip patients with questions that increase their likelihood of being informed about and involved in their care. These questions are: (1) What is my main problem? (2) What do I need to do? and (3) Why is it important for me to do this? Being prepared with these and other questions can help patients get the most appropriate treatment, complete information, and positive assurance. More specifically, such questions can be used or adapted to find out when and how treatments are relevant to a patient's gender transition.

CONCLUSION

A trans individual's health goes beyond simply showing up to the doctor's office. The decisions made in health care carry over into a trans patient's personal and social life, and vice versa. Therefore, the separate identities a trans individual holds (social, personal, and health) are intertwined and reciprocal. The interaction of these identities is easily seen in the doctor's office. We position individuals as cultural beings who bring their personal identities, social identities, and cultural experiences into the doctor's office. This biopsychosocial approach takes into consideration various factors of a person's life (physical, environmental, emotional, spiritual, and social) that contribute positively and negatively to his or her health. As evident in the themes found in this study, the biopsychosocial model is an effective framework of health care for trans individuals. When all aspects of an individual's health are considered, all parties involved experience satisfaction. Our recommendations to health professionals are modeled after the biopsychosocial model and aim to improve health care for all trans individuals by suggesting these professionals use the biopsychosocial model to help understand a trans individual's full health.

II

ACCESS, DISPARITIES, AND HARASSMENT UNDER THE GUISE OF POLICIES

Health Insurance Coverage for Same-Sex Couples

Disparities and Trends under DOMA

Gilbert Gonzales, Ryan Moltz, and Miriam King

$\mathcal{D}$isparities in health status, health behaviors, and health care access on the basis of sexual orientation have been largely ignored by researchers until recently. Literature reviews in public health, medicine, and nursing note a dearth of studies relating to the lesbian, gay, bisexual, and transgender (LGBT) population and report a disproportionate focus on HIV/AIDS and other sexually transmitted diseases (Boehmer, 2002; Snyder, 2011; Johnson, Smyer, & Yucha, 2012). Meanwhile, inequities in health care on the basis of sexual orientation were recently recognized by health policy makers as a public health priority and targeted for elimination (Institute of Medicine, 2011). For example, Healthy People 2020 goals, set by the U.S. federal government to monitor improvements in population health, now include improving "the health, safety, and well-being of lesbian, gay, bisexual, and transgender (LGBT) individuals" (United States Department of Health and Human Services, 2010).

Access to health insurance is a key area in which the LGB[1] population has been disadvantaged because same-sex couples face structural and policy barriers to adding their spouses and unmarried partners to employer-sponsored health insurance, the main source of health insurance for the nonelderly population in the United States (State Health Access Data Assistance Center, 2013). This chapter describes how health insurance coverage for nonelderly same-sex couples differs from coverage for different-sex couples and how coverage has changed over time. Before presenting the results of our research, we review legal barriers and findings from previous studies.

LEGAL BARRIERS TO INSURANCE COVERAGE

At the time of this writing, thirteen states and the District of Columbia recognize legal marriages for same-sex couples; six states extend civil unions or domestic partnerships to same-sex couples; and nearly all the remaining states ban same-sex marriage through legislative action or through amendments to their state constitutions (Human Rights Campaign, 2013b). The legal recognition of same-sex unions grants partnered LGB people numerous rights and benefits enjoyed by married different-sex couples. Although many benefits contingent on marital status are offered through federal and state governments in the form of taxation relief (Human Rights Campaign, 2013c), same-sex couples may also enjoy expanded private benefits through employment (United States General Accounting Office, 1997). When states enact same-sex marriage or civil unions that extend equal rights and protections to same-sex couples, *"fully insured"* private employers, who fall under the jurisdiction of state insurance regulators, are often required to treat married same-sex couples like married different-sex couples (Badgett, 2010). Fully insured employers are typically smaller firms that choose to provide health benefits to their employees through insurance companies (e.g., the firms and employees pay premiums to an insurer who manages the health plan and the financial risk). Most employees offered private insurance (approximately 58 percent); however, they maintain coverage through *"self-insured"* plans, or employer health plans whereby the employer takes on the financial risk rather than an insurance company (Crimmel, 2011). Self-insured plans are more common among larger employers and are regulated under the federal Employee Retirement Income Security Act (ERISA).

Until Section 3 of the federal Defense of Marriage Act (DOMA) was ruled unconstitutional in *United States v. Windsor* by the Supreme Court in June 2013, DOMA created additional barriers at the national level for all LGB workers interested in adding their spouses to employer-sponsored insurance (ESI). Section three of DOMA defined marriage as "a legal union between one man and one woman as husband and wife" for federal purposes like taxes on incomes, retirement and pension plans, and employer-sponsored health insurance (Defense of Marriage Act, 1996). Although the federal government does not tax employer contributions to a spouse's health benefits, a same-sex partner's health benefits were taxed under DOMA as if the employer contribution was taxable income. LGB employees paid on average $1,069 in additional federal income taxes when they added their same-sex spouses or partners to employer health plans (Badgett, 2007).[2] Given the limited reach of state policies that recognize same-sex relationships and the added federal barriers to adding a same-sex partner to a worker's employer-sponsored insurance under DOMA, disparities in health insurance coverage were thus expected.

PREVIOUS RESEARCH

Studying health insurance coverage in the LGB population is challenging because few nationally representative surveys collect information on sexual orientation.[3] Even though surveys generally do not ascertain sexual orientation, same-sex couples are identifiable in some nationally representative survey data based on information regarding the relationship of household members to the household reference person (sometimes called the "household head"); same-sex couples are identified when a person of the same sex as the household head is reported to be the head's "spouse" or "unmarried partner." Four previous studies have used intrahousehold information from federal surveys to compare health insurance coverage between individuals in same-sex relationships to couples in different-sex relationships.

Heck, Sell, and Gorrin (2006) used the National Health Interview Survey (NHIS) to compare health insurance coverage between individuals in same-sex relationships and married adults in different-sex relationships. The study found women in same-sex relationships were significantly less likely than married women in different-sex relationships to have health insurance, but health insurance coverage was not statistically different between men in same-sex relationships and married men in different-sex relationships. Ash and Badgett (2006) took advantage of larger samples in the Current Population Survey (CPS) and found that both men and women in same-sex couples were two to three times more likely to be uninsured than married people in different-sex relationships. Buchmueller and Carpenter (2010) used a national sample of adults aged twenty-five to sixty-four in the Behavioral Risk Surveillance System (BRFSS) to compare health insurance for co-resident persons in same-sex relationships versus those in different-sex relationships (both married and unmarried). Married adults in different-sex relationships had the highest rates and odds of health insurance coverage, followed by men and women in same-sex relationships, and then by unmarried men and women in different-sex relationships. Finally, Gonzales and Blewett (forthcoming) demonstrated that nonelderly same-sex couples in the 2008–2010 American Community Surveys (ACS) were less likely than their married counterparts in different-sex relationships to have health insurance through an employer in nearly every state. The largest disparities in ESI coverage for men were found in the South, while the largest disparities for women were found in the Midwest.

REVERSING DISPARITIES IN HEALTH INSURANCE

Despite these four studies indicating point-in-time disparities in health insurance and access to health care, employer surveys have indicated growing willingness among businesses to offer health benefits to same-sex partners. A survey of about 3,000 employers by the Mercer consulting firm reported that almost half (47 percent) of all large private firms (those with more than 500 employees) offered same-sex domestic partner benefits in 2012, compared to 39 percent in 2010 (Mercer, 2012). Coverage of same-sex partners varied widely by region, with firms in the Western United States reporting the highest offer rates (73 percent) and firms in the South reporting the lowest (30 percent). Similarly, according to the 2012 Employer Health Benefits Survey sponsored by the Kaiser Family Foundation and the Health Research and Educational Trust, almost half (42 percent) of large employers with 200 or more employees offer health benefits to same-sex domestic partners. Among all employers surveyed in the Kaiser study, 31 percent offered health benefits to same-sex domestic partners in 2012, up from 22 percent in 2008 (Claxton et al., 2012). Surveys by the Human Rights Campaign found that 62 percent of Fortune 500 companies offered equivalent medical benefits between spouses and same-sex domestic partners in 2013, up from 34 percent in 2002 (Human Rights Campaign 2002; Human Rights Campaign 2013d).[4]

Despite the state- and company-level efforts to reduce disparities in health insurance coverage for same-sex couples, many LGB people were likely to remain or become uninsured. Even when domestic partner benefits were available, some LGB employees may not have enrolled their partners in health plans because they preferred not to "come out" in their workplace or because of cost issues, including federal taxation of these benefits. Meanwhile, the growing number of employers offering domestic partner benefits during the past decade coincided with a general decline in the number of firms offering and the number of people covered by employer-sponsored insurance overall (Holahan & Cook, 2008; Holahan, 2010). The percentage of all people under age sixty-five with private health insurance declined steadily after 1980, from 79 percent in 1980 to 67 percent in 2007 (Cohen et al., 2009).

Although disparities in health insurance coverage are well documented for LGB Americans, much less is known about changes over time and recent developments following the expanded recognition of same-sex unions and same-sex partner benefits. We use data from the nation's leading source on population health, the National Health Interview Survey, to inform: (1) trends in health insurance coverage among same-sex couples compared to different-sex couples and (2) the relationship between being in a same-sex union versus an unmarried partnership and insurance coverage.

DATA AND METHODS

The National Health Interview Survey (NHIS) is a nationally representative household survey of the civilian noninstitutionalized population in the United States and has been conducted every year since 1957 by the National Center for Health Statistics (NCHS), an agency within the Centers for Disease Control and Prevention (CDC). To simplify pooling data across samples, we used the version of the NHIS data disseminated through the Integrated Health Interview Series (www.ihis.us), created by researchers at the Minnesota Population Center (2012). As mentioned above, NHIS data have been used before, by Heck et al. (2006), to study health insurance coverage for persons in same-sex couples, but we extend the time frame of our analysis (to include 1997 through 2012) and investigate the relationship between union status and health insurance coverage.

Prior to 2013, the NHIS did not collect information on sexual orientation. In our study, same-sex couples were identified when another person in the household was reported as the husband, wife, or unmarried partner of the household reference person and was the same sex as the reference person. Under DOMA, the U.S. Decennial Census and other surveys conducted by the Census Bureau (such as the ACS and CPS) have recoded same-sex spouses identified by husband or wife categories to unmarried partners (O'Connell & Gooding, 2007). Fortunately, the NCHS preserves these original "spouse" versus "unmarried partner" responses for same-sex couples in the NHIS. By pooling data from 1997 through 2012, we created a data set of 538,700 non-elderly adults between eighteen and sixty-four years of age and differentiated by relationship type: different-sex unmarried partners (n=56,807), same-sex unmarried partners (n=4,005), different-sex married spouses (n=487,561), and same-sex married spouses (n=667).

NHIS data provide rich detail on the type(s) of insurance coverage for people who have health insurance. In our analysis, each observation was assigned to having insurance through: (1) an employer or the military (as the policyholder or dependent); (2) directly purchased from an insurance company; (3) public programs, such as Medicaid and Medicare; or was (4) uninsured. For the purposes of this study, we assigned a "primary source" of health insurance coverage to people who reported multiple sources of coverage. Medicare was always considered the primary source of coverage, followed in our hierarchy by employer-sponsored insurance (ESI) or military health insurance (VA health insurance, TRICARE or CHAMPVA), Medicaid or other state programs, and directly purchased insurance. Individuals with ESI or military insurance were separated based on having insurance in their own name or having insurance through someone else's health plan as a dependent.

We defined individuals as uninsured if they had no reported insurance coverage or had only single-service coverage (such as dental insurance) or health care through the Indian Health Service, as these types of insurance and health care programs may not include comprehensive care to people enrolled (U.S. Census Bureau, 2013; National Center for Health Statistics, 2012a).

Our formal analysis consists of three parts. First, we document trends in uninsurance by relationship type to determine whether health insurance coverage has improved for men and women in same-sex relationships between 1997 and 2012. Estimates were pooled into four-year periods to support sufficient sample sizes. Second, we explore the distributional changes in types of health insurance coverage over time. We used a two-tailed test to determine differences in coverage types between the beginning period (1997–2000) and final period (2009–2012) of our time frame. For instance, we tested whether the percent of adults with ESI decreased between 1997–2000 and 2009–2012. Third, we estimate a multivariate logistic regression model to determine the relationship between being in a same-sex couple and having health insurance coverage in 1997–2000 versus in 2009–2012. We grouped together all persons in same-sex couples for 1997–2000, as no states legally recognized same-sex marriage during this period and few respondents referred to their same-sex partners as a husband or wife. We separated same-sex couples into two categories, married spouses and unmarried partners, for our analysis of 2009–2012 data. By these later years, some states legally recognized same-sex marriage, and more persons in same-sex couples reported their relationship as a husband or wife. In addition, by the end of the period, NHIS interviewers confirmed the accuracy of responses on relationship type and sex when someone was reported as a same-sex spouse of the household reference person. This minimizes the likelihood that same-sex married persons in our sample for 2009–2012 are actually miscoded different-sex married persons. Thus, for the most recent data, we evaluated whether being in a self-reported married same-sex relationship (rather than an unmarried same-sex partnership) affected the odds of lacking insurance.

We used the following logistic regression model on the entire sample to control for factors associated with health insurance coverage:

$$\text{Uninsurance} = \alpha + \beta_1 \text{Relationship}_i + \beta_k X_i + \varepsilon$$

Uninsurance represents the odds ratio of lacking any type of health insurance (relative to having health insurance coverage). *Relationship* indexes the type of relationship (married same-sex spouse, unmarried same-sex partner, or unmarried different-sex partner; married different-sex is the reference category). X indicates the vector of control variables, including:

- Age category (18–24, 25–34, 35–44, and 45–54; 55–64 is the reference group);
- Race and ethnicity (Hispanic, non-Hispanic Black, non-Hispanic other and multiple races; non-Hispanic White is the reference group);
- Educational attainment (less than high school, high school, and some college; college degree is the reference group);
- Family income (0–99 percent of the Federal Poverty Level [FPL], 101–199 percent FPL, 200–399 percent FPL; 400 percent FPL or more is the reference group);
- Employment status (part-time employment, unemployed, not in labor force; full-time employment was the reference group);
- Health status (excellent, very good, and good; fair/poor is the reference group);
- Region (Midwest, South, and West; Northeast is the reference group); and
- Presence of a biological, adopted, or stepchild under age eighteen.

Our model was estimated separately for men and women, first for the period 1997–2000 and then for 2009–2012. All regression models and coverage estimates were conducted using Stata 12 with survey weights adjusted for pooled estimation. Standard errors were calculated using Taylor linearized series. Because a large share of NHIS respondents does not report their income, we used the income variables with multiple imputation of missing data that were developed by the National Center for Health Statistics (2012b).[5]

TRENDS IN UNINSURANCE, 1997–2012

The percent of nonelderly adults lacking insurance coverage increased after 1997 for almost every relationship type (see Figure 5.1). Married persons in different-sex relationships were the least likely to be uninsured, with 12 percent lacking coverage in 1997–2000. That figure steadily rose to 14 percent by 2009–2012. Different-sex unmarried partners had the highest rates of uninsurance at 32 percent in 1997–2000 and 34 percent by the end of the period. Levels of uninsurance for men and women in same-sex relationships occupied a middle ground between married and unmarried different-sex couples and diverged by sex at the end of our study period. Uninsurance among women in same-sex relationships declined from 20 percent in 1997–2000 to 18 percent in 2009–2012. For men in same-sex relationships, uninsurance dropped from 21 percent in 1997–2000 to 18 percent in 2005–2008, then rose to 24 percent

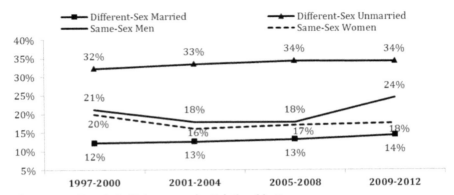

Figure 5.1.   Trends in Uninsurance by Relationship Type
Source: Authors' analysis of the National Health Interview Survey, 1997–2012.

in 2009–2012. Thus, women in same-sex relationships were the only group to experience a decline in uninsurance between 1997 and 2012.

TYPES OF HEALTH INSURANCE COVERAGE, 1997–2012

The types of health insurance coverage for men and women in same-sex relationships are presented in figures 5.2 and 5.3, respectively. In these figures we used a two-tailed test to determine whether there were significant differences in the distribution of insurance types between 1997–2000 and 2009–2012. As a comparison, we report the distribution of health insurance types for adults in married different-sex relationships in the appendix.

Consistent with increases in uninsurance, men in same-sex relationships were less likely to be policy holders of an employer-sponsored insurance (ESI) plan in 2009–2012 (50 percent) than in 1997–2000 (58 percent). The per-

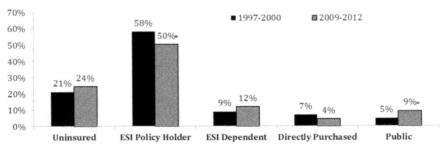

Figure 5.2.   Types of Health Insurance for Men in Same-Sex Relationships
Source: Authors' analysis of the National Health Interview Survey, 1997–2012.

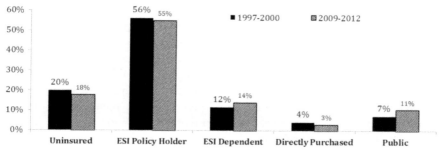

Figure 5.3.   Types of Health Insurance for Women in Same-Sex Relationships
Source: Authors' analysis of the National Health Interview Survey, 1997–2012.

centage of men in same-sex relationships who were dependents on another person's ESI plan increased, however, from 9 percent to 12 percent, though this increase was not statistically significant. The percentage of men with health insurance directly purchased from an insurance company also declined, from 7 percent to 4 percent, while public coverage increased from 5 percent to 9 percent. When married men in different-sex relationships were used as a comparison group (appendix 4.1), we found similar changes in health insurance coverage, including a decline in the percent who were ESI policyholders (from 60 percent in 1997–2000 to 55 percent in 2009–12) and increasing utilization of public insurance (from 4 percent to 7 percent). Notably, there were no differences in coverage as dependents on another person's ESI plan (consistently 19 percent) or in directly purchased insurance (consistently 4 percent) for men in different-sex marriages.

Although men in same-sex couples and different-sex marriages experienced worsening health insurance coverage since the late 1990s, this was partly offset by growing reliance on dependent coverage through employment-based plans for men in same-sex relationships. Increasing rates of dependent coverage for men in same-sex relationships are consistent with growing legal recognition of same-sex unions at the state level and increasing offer rates of domestic partner benefits by employers.

Women in same-sex relationships did not experience a statistically significant decline in ESI coverage (56 percent in 1997–2000 versus 55 percent in 2009–2012; Figure 5.3). The percentage with ESI as a dependent increased from 12 percent in 1997–2000 to 14 percent in 2009–2012, though this change was not statistically significant. Women in same-sex relationships with health insurance directly purchased from an insurance company dropped from a 4 percent coverage rate in 1997–2000 to a 3 percent coverage rate in 2009–2012. The percentage with public health insurance increased from 7 percent to 11 percent. Unlike their counterparts in same-sex relationships, women in married different-sex relationships exhibited increased uninsurance rates, for unin-surance increased by 2 percentage points for this group between 1997–2000 and 2009–2012 (appendix 4.2). The percentage who were ESI policyholders rose slightly (from 29 percent in 1997–2000 to 34 percent in 2009–2012); the percentage who were dependents on a husband's ESI health plan dropped sub-stantially (from 49 percent down to 40 percent). For this comparison group, reliance on public insurance rose (from 4 percent to 8 percent), while directly purchased insurance did not change (consistently 5 percent).

Observed estimates of insurance coverage over time indicate that women in same-sex relationships were able to capitalize on growing legal recognition and domestic partner benefits, by maintaining insurance coverage as depen-dents on ESI plans, while their counterparts in married different-sex relation-ships experienced substantial declines in dependent coverage.

Notably, both men and women in same-sex relationships experienced much lower levels of dependent coverage than people in married different-sex relationships. Approximately 11 percent and 14 percent of men and women in same-sex relationships, respectively, reported health insurance through an employer as a dependent. In contrast, 19 percent and 40 percent of men and women in married different-sex relationships reported having health insurance through an employer as a dependent.

MULTIVARIATE ANALYSIS

Although the trend analyses presented above demonstrated that persons in same-sex relationships and unmarried different-sex partnerships were more likely to be uninsured than their married different-sex counterparts, the ob-served estimates did not control for known differences between people in these various union types (Carpenter & Gates, 2008). Unmarried different-sex partners tend to be younger and are more likely to be poor than their married counterparts. Lower levels of socioeconomic status subsequently translate into lower levels of health insurance coverage. Persons in same-sex relationships, however, are more likely to report higher incomes and more education than those in different sex unions (Black, Sanders, & Taylor, 2007; Carpenter & Gates, 2008). As expected, the same-sex couples in our NHIS data reported high levels of socioeconomic status (appendix 4.3). Nonelderly men in same-sex relationships were more likely than men in different-sex couples to have a college degree (45.7 percent) and report an income over 400 percent of the federal poverty level (65.1 percent), which was $44,680 for an individual and $92,200 for a family of four in 2012.[6] The percent that were employed full-time was similar for men in same-sex and different-sex relationships.

The women in same-sex relationships included in our sample also ex-hibited high levels of socioeconomic status based on education, income, and employment. Almost 42 percent had a college degree, a figure much higher than the 31 percent and 19 percent of married and unmarried women in different-sex relationships. Women in same-sex couples had the highest levels of full-time employment (67.2 percent) and incomes above 400 percent of the poverty level (54.8 percent). Like their male counterparts, women in *unmarried* different-sex relationships were least likely to have college degrees and more likely to be living in poverty (<100 percent FPL) or near poverty (100–200 percent FPL). In this section, we test whether disparities in health insurance persisted over time after controlling for demographic and economic charac-teristics that contribute to whether a person has insurance. We also document whether being in a married relationship versus an unmarried partnership influ-enced health insurance coverage for same-sex couples. We do not distinguish married from unmarried same-sex couples in the early period (1997–2000), but we do separate same-sex married persons in analyses for 2009–2012. Although no states legally recognized same-sex marriage in the early portion of our study (1997–2000), eight states and the District of Columbia recognized same-sex marriages by the end of our study period (2009–2012), while seven other states legally recognized same-sex "civil unions" or "domestic partnerships."[7]

At the beginning of our study period in 1997–2000, men in unmarried different-sex relationships (odds ratio [OR]=2.81) and men in same-sex rela-tionships (OR=2.65) were more likely to be uninsured than men in married different-sex relationships (table 5.1). By the end of the study period (2009–2012), men in unmarried different-sex and unmarried same-sex relationships continued to experience greater odds (OR=2.24 and OR=3.14, respectively) of lacking health insurance than men in married different-sex couples. Strik-ingly, men that reported being in *married* same-sex relationships were statisti-cally not any more likely to be uninsured than their married counterparts in different-sex relationships (OR=1.71).

A very similar pattern was found among women. Prior to any legal rec-ognition of same-sex marriage in the pooled period 1997–2000, both women in unmarried different-sex relationships (OR=2.29) and women in same-sex relationships (OR=2.98) were more likely to be uninsured than women in married different-sex relationships. By 2009–2012, disparities in insurance coverage persisted for women in unmarried different-sex relationships and unmarried same-sex relationships (OR=1.78 and OR=1.71, respectively). Disparities in health insurance coverage were not statistically significant for married women in same-sex relationships (OR=1.34).

Although uninsurance for same-sex couples is lower than for unmar-ried different-sex partners in the trend data shown in figures 5.2 and 5.3, the

Table 5.1. Adjusted Odds Ratio of Being Uninsured, by Union Status

	Men				Women			
	1997–2000	n	2009–2012	n	1997–2000	n	2009–2012	n
Different-Sex, Married	Ref.	66,616	Ref.	57,907	Ref.	69,729	Ref.	61,171
Different-Sex, Unmarried	2.81**	6,446	2.24**	8,638	2.29**	6,512	1.78**	8,760
Same-Sex, Married	—	—	1.71	62	—	—	1.34	86
Same-Sex, Unmarried	2.65**	454	3.14**	620	2.98**	371	1.71**	705

Note: Adjusted for age, race and ethnicity, education, poverty status, employment, region, presence of a child in household, health status, and year. *p<0.05, **p<0.01

Source: Integrated Health Interview Series, 1997–2012.

adjusted odds ratios for uninsurance for same-sex partners are higher in our multivariate models. This shift occurs because the high socioeconomic levels of partnered LGB persons predict greater insurance coverage than is actually occurring. Without legal recognition of same-sex relationships at the state and federal level, socioeconomic advantage in terms of full-time employment, education, and income does not yield the expected level of insurance coverage for those in same-sex relationships.

DISCUSSION

Our study highlights how partnered sexual minorities have historically experienced barriers to adding their partners to health insurance through employers. We found nonelderly men and women in same-sex relationships were more likely to be uninsured under the Defense of Marriage Act (DOMA) and less likely to have employer-sponsored insurance (ESI) as a dependent than adults in married different-sex relationships. Over the past decade, some states have adopted policies that recognize same-sex unions and made it easier for same-sex couples to add their partners to ESI plans, but federal laws prevented many same-sex couples from doing so.

The U.S. Supreme Court recently recognized this obstacle when it struck down Section 3 of DOMA in *United States v. Windsor* and affirmed leaving the definition of marriage to states. In writing for the opinion of the Court, Justice Anthony Kennedy agreed that Section 3 directly inhibited access to health insurance: "By its great reach, DOMA touches many aspects of married and family life, from the mundane to the profound. It prevents same-sex married couples from obtaining government health benefits they would otherwise receive. . . . It raises the cost of health care for families by taxing health benefits provided by employers to their workers' same-sex spouses" (*United States v. Windsor*, 2013, p 23–24). Based on this ruling, married same-sex couples residing in states with legal same-sex marriage will find it easier to add their spouses to ESI plans, whereas same-sex couples in other states will continue to experience state-level barriers to ESI comparable to DOMA.

Our study also detects early evidence of this bifurcated treatment, for our results demonstrated that uninsurance disparities were narrower and not statistically significant for *married* same-sex couples but persisted for *unmarried* same-sex couples in 2009–2012. The advantage enjoyed by married same-sex couples in our data preceded the *United States v. Windsor* decision, and it suggests that state laws recognizing same-sex marriage (or civil unions) reduced barriers to insurance coverage to some extent. Married same-sex couples in states recognizing their marriages may enjoy further gains in insurance coverage and access to health care following *US v. Windsor*, while the absence of legally recognized unions in other states may widen health care disparities within the LGB population. Much depends on how rapidly same-sex marriage extends to other states, now that support for same-sex marriage outweighs opposition in national opinion polls.[8]

Meanwhile, many private employers are ahead of the game, for growing numbers of employers, and especially larger companies, already offer domestic partner benefits to attract and retain a diverse and talented workforce. Indeed, when we stratify our analysis of insurance coverage by firm size for the randomly selected sample adult in each couple type, we find more adults in same-sex relationships are covered by ESI when the sample adult works for a company with more than fifty employees (77 percent in 2009–2012) than when the sample adult works for a company with fewer than fifty employees (56 percent in 2009–2012; figure 5.4).[9] Although a positive relationship between insurance coverage and firm size is expected, more notable is the smaller disparity between same-sex couples and married different-sex couples in larger firms. The differences in ESI coverage exceed 10–15 percent among smaller firms, whereas the differences fall between 6 percent and 9 percent in firms with more than fifty employees. Despite these important gains, however, our results indicate that both married or unmarried same-sex couples still have a long way to go to reach equity in insurance coverage, compared to their married counterparts in different-sex relationships.

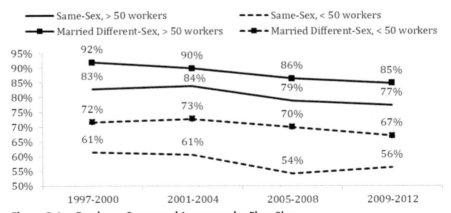

Figure 5.4.   Employer-Sponsored Insurance by Firm Size
Source: Authors' analysis of the National Health Interview Survey, 1997–2012.

LIMITATIONS

There are several limitations to conducting couple-based studies in LGB health research that should be acknowledged (Carpenter & Gates, 2008; Gates & Steinberger, 2009; O'Connell & Feliz, 2011; Bates, DeMaio, Robins, & Hicks, 2012). Health researchers and demographers are concerned with data quality when joining relationship information and the sex of individual household members to identify same-sex couples. Misreporting sex among married different-sex couples, although not common, may unintentionally include heterosexual couples as "false positives" among same-sex partners (Gates & Steinberger, 2009; O'Connell & Feliz, 2011). This is especially challenging when studying small populations like LGB persons. Even if a small portion of different-sex couples misreport gender, the result could lead to a cumbersome number of false positives in our already-small sample of same-sex couples. As a precautionary measure, we confirmed that our trend analyses in figures 5.1–5.3 are consistent with or without including potentially "false positive" same-sex married couples.

Beginning in 2011, National Health Interview Survey interviewers routinely asked follow-up questions to confirm the accuracy of the reported relationship and gender of any person recorded as the same-sex spouse of the household head. Although we use small sample sizes for our multivariate analysis (see table 5.1), the number of reported same-sex married persons for the immediately preceding years is similar to the benchmark 2011 figure. Other elements contributing to the accuracy of the NHIS data include the use of experienced and well-trained interviewers asking face-to-face questions during a household visit and confirmation of the sex of the randomly selected sample adult later in the interview.[10] Weighing these various factors, we assume that unions involving same-sex "spouses" in 2009–2012 generally had some level of legal recognition or were reported by couples that perceived their relationships as marriages rather than partnerships. Therefore, we classified these couples identified at the end of the period as "same-sex married" but the label may capture factors beyond legal standing. Partnered sexual minorities may report themselves as married if their marriages are authorized by their state of residence, if they have been together for a longer duration, or if they equate their relationship to a marriage even when their state government does not (Bates et al., 2012). These couples may be more stable or more willing to publicly announce their relationship to employers and request dependent coverage for their spouses.

Finally, findings based on LGB couples cannot be generalized to the entire LGB population. Levels of uninsurance are potentially greater for LGB people not captured in our analysis. Single, nonelderly LGB adults or LGB adults in early and less stable relationships, for instance, rely on their own employers for health insurance. Additionally, selection bias may affect whether and how same-sex couples identify themselves. Partnered sexual minorities are more likely to be white and highly educated, compared to nonpartnered sexual minorities (Carpenter & Gates, 2008). As noted, our sample of same-sex couples are highly educated, more likely to work full-time, and have incomes over 400 percent FPL, all factors associated with having insurance coverage as an employment benefit.

Fortunately, the amount of nationally representative data on the LGBT population can be expected to increase in the near future. The overturning of DOMA means that large federal surveys such as the American Community Survey and the Current Population Survey will likely stop obscuring differences by union type through automatically recoding all self-reported same-sex spouses as "unmarried partners." Beginning with the 2013 National Health Interview Survey (NHIS), all sample adults will be asked if they view themselves as gay, straight, bisexual, or something else (United States Department of Health and Human Services, 2011). This new information will support research on people who self-identify as LGB whether in a partnership or not. Additional research should investigate disparities in health insurance among single LGB people and continue to explore how partnership affects not only health insurance but also additional issues in accessing health care such as finding providers and affording health care costs. Responses to sexual orientation questions will likely remain sensitive in many parts of the country, though, for many LGBT persons may choose not to disclose their sexual orientation. Relatedly, some people who engage in same-sex sexual behavior may not self-identify as being gay or lesbian.

CONCLUSIONS

One by one, states are passing legislation to guarantee to people in committed same-sex relationships the legal right to marry and enjoy the benefits that accrue to married couples. Our findings indicate that general declines in the availability of employer-sponsored health insurance coverage increased levels of uninsurance since 1997 for nonelderly adults in all types of unions, including different-sex marriages, different-sex unmarried partnerships, and same-sex unions. Partially countering this negative trend were some gains in employment-based dependent coverage for persons in same-sex relationships, increased offering of domestic partner benefits by employers (especially in

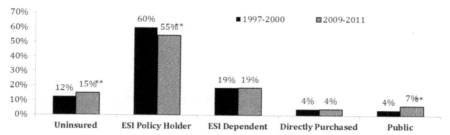

Figure 5.5.   Types of Health Insurance for Men in Different-Sex Married Relationships
Source: Authors' analysis of the National Health Interview Survey, 1997–2012.

large firms), and reduced disparities in insurance coverage for same-sex married persons by 2009–2012.

Even though thirteen states and the District of Columbia have adopted marriage equality laws, most states continue to limit the rights of same-sex couples. Following the recent decisions by the U.S. Supreme Court in 2013, some federal barriers to adding same-sex partners to employer-sponsored health insurance, such as taxing health insurance plans for dependent same-sex spouses, were removed for married persons in states legalizing same-sex marriage. Similarly, federal employees, including members of the Armed Services and legislative employees living in states recognizing same-sex marriage, have now gained access to health insurance benefits for their same-sex legally married spouses. Disparities in health insurance are likely to persist or broaden in the short-term, especially in states without legal same-sex marriage. To address these issues, state policy makers can persist in adopting same-sex marriage laws, and private employers can continue to voluntarily expand health insurance to same-sex spouses and partners.

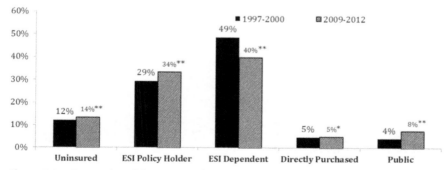

Figure 5.6.   Types of Health Insurance for Women in Different-Sex Married Relationships
Source: Authors' analysis of the National Health Interview Survey, 1997–2012.

Table 5.2. Sample Descriptive Statistics, by Relationship Type: National Health Interview Survey, 1997–2012

	Men			Women		
	Same-Sex Couples	Different-Sex Married	Different-Sex Unmarried	Same-Sex Married	Different-Sex Married	Different-Sex Unmarried
Education						
Less than high school	6.4%	12.6%	19.0%	6.5%	10.9%	16.2%
High school degree or GED	19.1%	28.1%	36.6%	21.0%	28.3%	32.1%
Some college or vocational	28.7%	26.6%	27.5%	30.3%	29.8%	32.6%
College degree	45.7%	32.7%	16.9%	42.1%	31.1%	19.2%
Income relative to FPL						
<100	6.8%	6.9%	15.6%	7.2%	6.6%	15.1%
100–200	8.5%	13.5%	21.1%	12.8%	13.5%	20.9%
200–400	19.6%	29.6%	30.8%	25.2%	29.9%	30.9%
400+	65.1%	50.0%	32.5%	54.8%	50.0%	33.1%
Employment						
Full-time	68.8%	78.9%	69.2%	66.8%	46.5%	52.2%
Part-time	12.6%	8.0%	12.9%	15.0%	20.2%	19.3%
Unemployed	4.0%	2.7%	7.0%	3.6%	2.2%	6.1%
Not in labor force	14.6%	10.4%	10.9%	14.6%	31.1%	22.4%

Note: GED = general equivalency diploma. FPL = federal poverty level. Weighted means are for adults aged eighteen to sixty-four years.

NOTES

1. Insurance coverage for transgender persons is an important issue, but this issue is beyond the scope of this chapter since the data sources reviewed here do not identify transgender individuals.

2. In addition to the taxation of health insurance for same-sex couples, ERISA regulations under DOMA meant that self-insured employer health plans were not required to extend benefits to same-sex spouses, even when a state recognized same-sex marriage. DOMA also precluded health insurance coverage for same-sex partners of federal workers in the Federal Employees Health Benefits Program. Similarly, under DOMA, same-sex partners of members of the armed forces could not qualify for military health insurance benefits, even after the repeal of the "Don't Ask, Don't Tell" policy in 2011. Finally, the federal law requiring employers to give their former employees the opportunity to continue their health insurance coverage by paying a premium (COBRA) did not guarantee such extended coverage to a same-sex spouse under DOMA.

3. Federal health surveys that ascertain sexual orientation include the National Health and Nutrition Examination Survey (NHANES), the National Survey of Family Growth (NSFG), the General Social Survey (GSS, with data on sexual behavior), the National Longitudinal Study of Adolescent Health (Add Health), and some state supplemental questions in the Behavioral Risk Factor Surveillance Survey (BRFSS) and the Youth Risk Behavior Surveillance System (YRBSS). The California Health Interview Survey (CHIS) also includes questions on sexual orientation. In 2013, questions on sexual orientation were included in the U.S. National Health Interview Survey (NHIS) for the first time.

4. As same-sex marriage is legally recognized in a growing number of states, some employers who offer benefits to same-sex domestic partners may decide to restrict health insurance coverage to legally married spouses, covering both same-sex and different-sex marriages.

5. The Division of Health Interview Statistics of the National Center for Health Statistics announced the release of the public use data files for the 2012 NHIS on June 28, 2013. The release of the 2012 NHIS imputed income files is scheduled for later in 2013. Thus, for 2012 data only, we did not use imputed income variables.

6. Family income data in the NHIS should be largely comparable for persons in married couples and persons in unmarried partnerships, since NHIS interviewers prompt respondents to include income of the unmarried partner when choosing the income category that fits their family. Family income data across union types is less comparable in some other sources, such as the Current Population Survey and U.S. census, where income from various sources is asked for each individual and then summed across persons related by blood or marriage (but not those related by unmarried partnership) to produce a family income figure.

7. States legalizing same-sex marriages by the end of 2012 included: Massachusetts (2004), Connecticut (2008), Iowa (2009), Vermont (2009), New Hampshire (2010), New York (2011), Maine (2012), and Washington (2012). Same-sex marriage laws

did not take effect until December 6, 2012, for the state of Washington and until December 29, 2012, for Maine. Maryland passed legislation recognizing same-sex marriages in 2012, but the law did not take effect until January 1, 2013. Same-sex marriage became available in the District of Columbia in 2010. States with same-sex civil unions included: New Jersey (2007), Illinois (2011), and Hawaii (2012); states with same-sex domestic partnerships included: Oregon (2008), Nevada (2009), and Wisconsin (2009).

8. Using one projection model, Nate Silver (2013) concluded, "By 2016, however, voters in thirty-two states would be willing to vote in support of same-sex marriage, according to the model. And by 2020, voters in forty-four states would do so, assuming that same-sex marriage continues to gain support at roughly its previous rate."

9. Data on firm size, or number of employees in the workplace, is only available for one randomly-selected "sample adult" per family. We assign the firm size reported for the sample adult to each adult in the relationship.

10. We are less confident about the accuracy of the NHIS data on same-sex spouses for 2004–2006, due to an increase in the number of such cases for those years. We suspect this derives from a difference in data cleaning procedures at the National Center for Health Statistics for the 2004–2006 samples.

Carving Triangles into Squares

The Effects of LGBTQ-Stigma-Related Stressors during Youth, Adulthood, and Aging

Dawn L. Strongin, Marc J. Silva, and Fredrick Smiley

> *"Of all the forms of inequality, injustice in health care is the most shocking and inhumane."*
>
> —*Martin Luther King Jr.*

Lesbian, gay, bisexual, transgender, and questioning (LGBTQ) people are members of every community in the United States, and they embody all ages, races, ethnicities, socioeconomic strata, educational levels, professions, and religions. As is true for all individuals in a cultural group, they also represent a wide variety of perspectives and needs. Despite significant cross-sectional representation, LGBTQ individuals endure a disproportionate burden of chronic psychosocial stressors from systematic harassment and discrimination stemming from their stigmatized status in American culture. In turn, these stressors contribute to the erosion of sexual minorities' physical and mental health throughout their lives. Sexual minorities experience significantly higher rates of depression, anxiety, and chronic diseases than heterosexuals (Amadio, 2006; Becker, Gates, & Newson, 2004).

Following the 2003 congressional mandate's guidelines, the U.S. Department of Health and Human Services now submits an annual report to identify disparities in health care in the United States. The intention of the government report is to facilitate policy-making and program decisions to address current and future needs of systematically underserved groups based on race, color, nationality, age, or disability. However, sexual minority status was not included in data analyses until 2012, rendering LGBTQ individuals invisible in public policy discussions. This negligence masks an ever-widening health gap between LGBTQ people and the majority culture in all stages of typical development. This oversight also reflects the historical American perception that

LGBTQ people are not fully functioning citizens but rather individuals with moral, medical, or personal problems (Dilley, Simmons, Boysun, Pizacani, & Stark, 2010; Mustanski, Garofalo, & Emerson, 2010).

EFFECTS OF STRESS-RELATED SOCIAL STIGMA

Until recently, pervasive stigma-related stressors have not been considered the antecedent of psychiatric disorders and health problems (Meyer, 2003). The chronic stressors associated with heterosexism and gender conformity originate from both objective and subjective realities. Objective reality, or externalized stressors, can be viewed as independent of personal characteristics or identification with a stigmatized group, such as systematic discrimination. Subjective realities, or internalized stressors, include personal appraisals of this objective reality. For example, if faced with discrimination, a negative self-appraisal (e.g., shame) can lead to chronic health problems (Johnson, Carrico, Chesney, & Morin, 2008; Szymanski, Kashubeck-West, & Meyer, 2008).

Many Americans experience chronic stressors. Difficult relationships, traffic jams, and approaching deadlines are not immediate threats to a person's life but more like an ocean grinding a mountain into gravel over time. Continuous leakage of stress hormones partially suppresses the immune system and upsets neurochemical balance, causing a vulnerability to chronic disease, cancer, and psychiatric disorders (Vyas, Mitra, Rao, & Chattarji, 2002; Baum, Garofalo, & Yali, 2006). Social support effectively buffers individuals from the negative effects of chronic stress (Roth, Mefford, & Barchas, 1982). For example, healthy social bonds increase chemicals, such as serotonin, oxytocin, and endorphins, which promote a life-enhancing sense of well-being and boost the emotional and somatic resources needed to cope with stressors (Roth, Mefford, & Barchas; Young & Akil, 1985). Conversely, social isolation and rejection from the community creates anguish and illness. When an individual is a member of a stigmatized minority group, disharmony occurs between the marginalized individual and dominant culture.

The stressors associated with LBGTQ stigma compound the health effects of average stressors. Over time, the weight of these additional stressors further contributes to mental and/or physical decline and poor coping tools, such as higher rates of substance abuse (Human Rights Campaign, 2011) Approximately 20 percent to 30 percent of gay and transgender people report abusing substances, compared to 9 percent of the general population (National Survey of Substance Abuse Treatment Services, 2010; Hatzenbuehler, 2009). People who are both LGBTQ and members of a racial or ethnic minority will endure the highest levels of stigma-related stress (Diaz, Ayala, Bein, Henne,

& Marin, 2001; Cochran, Mays, Alegria, Ortega & Takeuchi, 2007). For instance, a gay African-American man faces stressors associated with racism and heterosexism combined, which in turn further compounds his stress load and health burden (Balsam, Molina, Beadnell, Simoni, & Walters, 2011).

Objective reality (i.e., discrimination and harassment), particularly in conjunction with a negative personal appraisal (i.e., shame and guilt), takes its toll on physical and mental health. However, the specific nature of sexual stigma has changed over time in the United States, reflecting perceptual shifts of sexual and gender identity in the dominant American culture. These changes have been mirrored in the many facets of LGBTQ stigma in the American psyche and result in specific problems for the stigmatized individual during various stages of typical development.

THE AMERICAN HISTORY OF LGBTQ STIGMA

"Don't walk in my head with your dirty feet."

—*Leo Buscaglia*

It is important to understand the evolution of stigma against LGBTQ people to appreciate how vestigial stigma-related beliefs influence American public consciousness about sexuality and gender, and in turn, destroy people's health and well-being. Contemporary attitudes toward homosexuality and gender identity are founded on a history of religious, legal, medical, and psychiatric views of sexuality (Bayer, 1987; Duberman, Vicinus, & Chauncey Jr., 1989). The variety of stigmatized attitudes toward sexual minorities derive from two schools of thought: (1) volitional breaking of moral and secular laws and (2) pathological manifestation of underlying medical or psychiatric conditions (Wilkerson, 1994). Although these perceptions and attitudes differ in terms of where to place blame, they foster the persistence of LGBTQ stigma in the United States to this present day (Mays & Cochran, 2001; Herek, 1990).

Sexual and gender identity first became a stigmatizing target when Puritans carried the concept with them from Britain to the American colonies. They left many of Britain's laws behind, with the exception of the Buggery Act, Britain's first secular law to criminalize anal penetration and bestiality (Hyde, 1970). The pairing of these disparate behaviors under one law established a revolting psychological link between (male) homosexual relationships and inhuman behavior. Before the arrival of the colonial settlers, most Native Americans held two-spirit, or transgender, people in high esteem for embodying the spirit of a man and the spirit of a woman (Williams, 1986).

In contrast, heretics and homosexuals were executed in the Puritanical New World (Bayer, 1987).

The conjoined sexual stigmas of sin and crime remained firmly rooted in American consciousness for five hundred years. An offshoot of this stigma grew when physicians and psychiatrists perceived homosexuality as a pathological disorder toward the end of the nineteenth century (Mays & Cochran, 2001; Hatzenbuehler, 2009). Austro-German psychiatrist Richard von Krafft-Ebing's belief that homosexuality was an inherited degeneracy influenced a generation of physicians, psychiatrists, and eugenicists (Ellis, 1915), as well as shifted blame (and stigma) from willful criminal behavior to a heritable pathological disorder:

> No legislation finds extramarital gratification of the sexual drive to be criminal in and of itself; the fact that the [sexual deviant] feels in a perverse manner is not his fault, but rather that of an abnormal natural constitution (Krafft-Ebing, 1886; in Ellis, 1915, p. 410).

Krafft-Ebing's view of heritability influenced physician Havelock Ellis, who believed homosexuals inherited opposite-sex traits, known as sexual inversion (Ellis, 1915). Contrary to Krafft-Ebing, however, Ellis did not perceive homosexuality as degenerate and in fact highlighted the overrepresentation of homosexuals who had achieved creative excellence. Following Havelock Ellis' example, Sigmund Freud believed that adult heterosexuals retain the homosexual component, albeit in sublimated form, and thus homosexuality itself can be neither criminal nor pathological. In 1935, Freud wrote a letter to an American mother who hoped psychoanalysis would cure her son:

> Homosexuality is assuredly no advantage, but it is nothing to be ashamed of, no vice, no degradation, it cannot be classified as an illness; we consider it to be a variation of the sexual function produced by a certain arrest of sexual development. Many highly respectable individuals of ancient and modern times have been homosexuals, several of the greatest men among them (Plato, Michelangelo, Leonardo da Vinci, etc.). It is a great injustice to persecute homosexuality as a crime, and cruelty too. . . . If [your son] is unhappy, neurotic, torn by conflicts, inhibited in his social life, analysis may bring him harmony, peace of mind, full efficiency whether he remains a homosexual or gets changed . . . (reprinted in Jones, 1957, 208–209).

Freud's assurances helped lift the burden of shame for American sexual minorities during the 1920s and early 1930s, permitting the homosexual subculture to thrive. By the mid 1930s, however, psychiatrists wrestled the controversy regarding the source of homosexuality back into the realm of pathology. Medically trained psychiatrists postulated that humans were innately bisexual, and appropriate social development guided individuals toward healthy heterosexual relationships (Bayer, 1987; Drescher, 1998). Homosexuality, therefore, was a pathological response to salient environmental experiences or obstacles that altered heterosexual development, such as early parental conflicts leading to phobic avoidance of the opposite sex (Rado, 1940; Lewes, 2009; Bayer; Drescher). Outpatient treatment included psychoanalysis. Intractable cases, however, were involuntarily hospitalized for treatments that included lobotomies, electroconvulsive therapy, and chemical castration (Minton, 2002; Milar, 2011). It was during this time that the epithet for homosexual, "fruitcake," became the epithet for insane, tying the homosexual stigma to insanity in popular culture (Kronemeyer, 1980). Resistance to involuntary hospitalization and treatment became an early focus for gay rights advocates (Fitzpatrick, 2004).

Most psychiatrists' knowledge of sexual minorities during this time was solely based on their clinical practices with maladjusted homosexual patients seeking therapeutic relief. Few clinicians had the opportunity to study sexual minorities who neither came for psychological help nor were found in mental hospitals, disciplinary barracks in the Armed Services, or in prison populations (Hooker, 1957). Hence, their clinical findings represented a skewed sample of homosexuals, and did not generalize to homosexuals who had not sought treatment or were not incarcerated for their sexual identities.

Declassification of Homosexuality by the American Psychiatric Association

The last half of the twentieth century marks the beginning of empirical studies used to uncouple pathology from sexual diversity. The American Psychiatric Association (APA) removed homosexuality from its diagnostic manual in 1973 after repeated evidence of well-adjusted sexual minorities (Hire, 2007). Until this time, the Cold War American psyche was threatened by a two-headed menace to American safety and decency: communism and homosexuality. Madison Avenue, Wall Street, and the White House cultivated fear during the Cold War and offered a solution every good American should undertake: compliance to rigid gender roles and heterosexist ideals. The heterosexual nuclear family offered the patriotic virtue needed to strengthen a nation under chronic atomic threat. Returning soldiers displaced Rosie the Riveter in the workplace, while Susie Homemaker raised the country's population boom (May, 1988; Cowan, 1983).

Psychiatrists supported the view that those who engaged in perverse (homosexual) behaviors were emotionally unstable and thus national security risks. Homosexual men were now seen as indecent, immoral, *and* un-American, while career women became unlovely, man-haters (Cowan, 1983).

President Eisenhower signed Executive Order 10450 in 1953, making it legal to conduct investigations of individuals suspected of "sexual perversities" (18 FR 2489, 3, CFR, 1949–1953). Over the next year and a half, 640 federal employees lost their jobs due to allegations of homosexuality, and countless state and local government employees were later fired as well (Fitzpatrick, 2004).

It was during this time that Indiana University-based sex researcher Alfred Kinsey published his findings on the prevalence of sexual diversity in the United States (Kinsey, Pomeroy, & Martin, 1948; Kinsey, Pomeroy, Martin, & Gebhard, 1953). The results astounded conservative America. Using in-depth, face-to-face interviews of more than 5,000 men and women each, Kinsey found that 10 percent of the men and 2 percent to 6 percent of the women reported only homosexual experiences, while 37 percent of men and 13 percent of women had at least one same-sex experience. Despite later discovery of the study's sampling bias (i.e., one-fourth of the male sample had been incarcerated, and 5 percent were male prostitutes), the 10 percent figure remained in the American consciousness. The concept that sexual diversity was normal found a foothold in American reality, and was reflected in later gay and civil rights movements during the 1960s and 1970s (Fitzpatrick, 2004).

Sputnik's 1957 Earth orbit motivated the United States to sharpen its scientific outlook in the latter part of the 1950s. During this time, American psychologist Evelyn Hooker's research was the first in a series of unbiased empirical studies comparing nonpsychiatric samples of hetero- and homosexual individuals (Hooker, 1957). Hooker asked experienced psychologists, unaware of the participants' sexual status, to interpret projective tests of thirty nonpatient heterosexual and thirty nonpatient homosexual men whose self-appraisals of their sexual identities were positive. These tests were chosen to determine the psychological well-being of the participants. The psychologists found no differences in the psychological well-being between the two groups. The study's findings strengthened the argument that self-appraisal of sexual identity directly affects health, disputing previous views of homosexuality as the manifestation of a pathological disorder.

Despite evidence that sexual minority status is not a pathological symptom, the stigmas of immorality and pathology continued to create unrelenting stigma-related stress for LGBTQ people. President Clinton repealed the Executive Order to eliminate sexual minorities from government employment in 1993; however, it was under the stipulation that LGBTQ military personnel remain closeted, commonly known as "Don't Ask, Don't Tell" (Streitmatter, 2009; Burroway, 2008). It was not until 2003 that the Supreme Court finally decriminalized adult consensual sex nationally, finally uncoupling legal from moral sanctions against sexual minority people in the United States (Mucciaroni, 2008; Human Rights Campaign, 2011).

IMPORTANCE OF CULTURAL COMPETENCY

"In times of stress, the best thing we can do for each other is to listen with our ears and our hearts and to be assured that our questions are just as important as our answers."

—*Fred Rogers*

Many times, our health care system distributes services inefficiently and unevenly across populations as some Americans receive worse care than others. These disparities may be due to differences in access to care, provider bias, poor provider-patient communication, or poor health literacy. For example, women and men in same-sex relationships were less likely have health insurance coverage, were less likely to have had a medical check up in the last year, and were more likely to report unmet medical needs, with LGBTQ people of color experiencing poorer health than their Caucasian counterparts (Buchmueller & Carpenter, 2010; Kim & Fredriksen-Goldsen, 2012). Many LGBTQ people often decline to seek health care in times of need out of fear of discrimination and poor treatment by health care professionals, or because of the fear that their medical records may contribute to work-related discrimination (Croteau, 1996).

The health disparities widen when age is taken into consideration. For example, LGBTQ youth report higher initial rates of substance use with increasing usage over time, compared to heterosexual youth (Marshall, Friedman, Stall, & Thompson, 2009). The adult LGBTQ population struggles with the consequences of legislation and discrimination (Croteau, 1996), while the aging LGBTQ population has had to manage the lasting effects of the AIDS epidemic and the effects of long-term discrimination. The stressors associated with each cohort are a direct result of societal stigmas.

Stressors Associated with LGBTQ Individuals

Adolescence. LBGTQ adolescents endure a disproportionate burden of stress compared to their heterosexual counterparts. Researchers have identified that they negotiate challenges and needs common to all teens, such as development of identity, intimacy, social and emotional well-being, and physical health (Cox, Dewaele, Van Houtte, & Vincke, 2011). However, their process of self-discovery and establishment of healthy relationships are confounded with coming to terms with rejection and/or retaliation related to their sexual identity. Consequently, LGBTQ youth have additional internal and external problems such as acceptance of sexual identity, "coming out," and dealing with minority stress (Cox et al.). As a result, LGBTQ adolescents are more vulnerable to risky coping behaviors, such as dropping out of school, drug abuse, suicidal ideation, depression, anxiety, and unprotected sex (Frankowski, 2004). LGBTQ youth, for example, are two times more likely to experiment with drugs and alcohol as compared with heterosexual youth (Human Rights Campaign, 2013a). The stressors that arise for LGBTQ adolescents begin with the first recognition of their sexual minority identity.

Identity as a Sexual Minority.   Many LGBTQ individuals become aware of their sexual minority status at an early age. The homophobia and stigma from society pave a grim path for people coming to terms with their sexual identity. Societal and familial judgments produce stressors not common to heterosexual adolescents. This year, the Human Rights Campaign investigated the stressors that most concern today's LGBTQ and heterosexual adolescents (Human Rights Campaign, 2013a). Participants were asked what they feared most and what they most wanted to change in their lives. The majority of LGBTQ adolescents reported greatest concern for their safety and security, even in their own homes. LGBTQ youth are twice as likely to be physically assaulted than heterosexual youth (Human Rights Campaign). Like all teens, LGBTQ adolescents worry about grades, finances, and their futures; these adolescents have additional anxiety about the life-altering matters that face them every day (Human Rights Campaign). Early LGBTQ positive mental health hinges on acceptance of their sexual identity. Rejection at the level of core identity makes disclosure one of the most difficult risks LGBTQ individuals can take.

Coming Out.   Disclosing LGBTQ identity to self and others most often occurs during adolescence. However, coming out is rarely a single event; rather, it is usually a lifelong process that parallels psychological and physical development. It is among the most difficult stressors for sexual minorities at any age, and particularly during adolescence. Today, LGBTQ teens are making the bold decision to come out at significantly earlier ages than previous generations. The national coming out age in 1991 was twenty-five years old; in 2010, it dropped to sixteen years old (Shilo & Savaya, 2011). Coming out during adolescence carries the risk of rejection from friends and family, possibility of homelessness, loss of financial support, and discrimination at school or work (Case Western Reserve University, 2013.). Some LGBTQ people wait until they are financially independent to disclose their sexual identities to anyone. Alan Downs (2005) vividly describes the terror young gay men may experience in his book, *The Velvet Rage:*

> Along with the growing knowledge that we were different was an equally expanding fear that our "different-ness" would cause us to lose the love and affection of our parents. This terror of being abandoned, alone, and unable

to survive forced us to find a way—any way—to retain our parent's love. We couldn't change ourselves, but we could change the way we acted. We could hide our differences, ingratiate ourselves to our mothers, and distance ourselves from our fathers whom we somehow knew would destroy us if he discovered our true nature (Downs, 2005, pp. 10–11).

Too many LGBTQ adolescents fear of rejection from family. Approximately 30 to 40 percent of homeless youths are sexual minorities (Goodenow, Szalacha, & Westheimer, 2006), and almost three-quarters of these youths report significantly more familial maltreatment and victimization at school as well (Goodenow, Szalacha, & Westheimer).

Victimization at School. Adolescent sexual minorities are three times more likely than heterosexuals to miss days at school in order to avoid persistent victimization by their peers, causing them to perform poorly academically (Kosciw, Palmer, Kull, & Greytak, 2013; Goodenow, Szalacha, & Westheimer, 2006). The perception of being a sexual minority can have damaging effects (Almeida, Johnson, Corliss, Molnar, & Azrael, 2009). Half of LGBTQ youths report they have been verbally harassed at school (Human Rights Campaign, 2011), with one in ten also withstanding physical assault at school. Transgender adolescents experience significantly more verbal and physical assault than lesbians, gay men, and bisexual people (Pilkington & D'Augelli, 1995; Cramer, McNiel, Holley, Shumway, & Boccellari, 2012).

Just as heterosexuals do, LGBTQ adolescents require acceptance and support to flourish. There are many steps schools can take to offer safer environments for LGBTQ adolescents and improve their learning environments. Supportive teachers and staff play the most important part to help LGBTQ adolescents feel comfortable at school and to reduce the rates of LGBTQ violence (Kosciw, Palmer, Kull, & Greytak, 2013). Student organizations, such as gay-straight alliances, help form friendships and a "queer-friendly" learning environment. Additionally, inclusive sexual education will give LGBTQ necessary information to make healthy decisions about their sexual behavior.

Sexual Education. Comprehensive sexual education gives all youth, despite sexual orientation or identity, the knowledge to develop healthy relationships and reduce their risks of acquiring sexually transmitted infections (National Coalition for LGBTQ Health, 2010). A significantly positive relationship exists between receiving sexual education at school and making healthy decisions about sexual behavior for heterosexual teens. Traditional sexual education is linked to postponement of sexual intercourse until fifteen years old and the use of birth control during the first sexual encounter (Orr, Beiter, & Ingersol, 1991; Mueller, Gavin, & Kulkarni, 2008). Adolescents learn the consequences of unprotected sex. The relationship between education and behavior is even more significant for at-risk racial minority teens. Racial minorities are more likely to engage in risky sexual behaviors to alleviate the cumulative burdens of racial stigma *and* adolescent stressors. For example, African American adolescent girls, who report hopelessness and depression, are at greatest risk for early sexual activity and unprotected sex (Orr, Beiter, & Ingersol). African American adolescent girls were 91 percent more likely to delay initiation of sexual intercourse until fifteen years old after receiving sexual education in school (Mueller, Gavin, Kulkarni). Sexual education teaches adolescents to consider the consequences of their sexual behaviors.

Despite sexual education's efficacy for heterosexual adolescents, courses that focus only on pregnancy prevention force LGBTQ adolescents to make uninformed decisions that may risk their health. Transgender adolescents are at the greatest disadvantage. Compared to males and females regardless of sexual orientation, transgender youth report the highest suicidal risk (Liu & Mustanski, 2012). Because little clinical or scientific information is available on transgender issues, these adolescents are especially vulnerable to poor health outcomes.

Sexual Behavior Health Risks.   LGBTQ adolescents learn about sexuality from a heterocentric perspective in sexual education courses. The most common types of sex education do not address the needs of sexual minorities; for example, abstinence-only education by definition excludes any notion that anyone may be other than heterosexual and provides no information about sexually-transmitted infection prevention (McGrath, 2004). Because sexual minority questions and issues are not addressed at school, they must rely on informal sources that may not offer correct information. For example, a common misconception among youth is that bisexual and lesbian women are not at risk for bacterial and viral infections (Skinner, Stokes, Kirlew, Kavanagh, & Forster, 1996). It is therefore important for physicians to inquire about sexual practices rather than orientation. In one instance, the term *lesbian* implies that a woman never has had sex with men, which may not be the case for every lesbian (Dolan & Davis, 2003). Another common misconception among adolescents is that two HIV-positive individuals can have unprotected sex with each other because they are already infected with HIV (Smith, Richman, & Little, 2005). Without sound sexual instruction, LGBTQ adolescents commonly seek information on Internet pornography sites, as early as eleven years old (Willingham, 2013). A popular trend in Internet pornography is *barebacking,* or unprotected anal sex. It is possible this trend has contributed to recent negative attitudes toward condom use by men who have sex with men (Shernoff, 2005). Many of the misconceptions and fallacies associated with high-risk sexual behavior can be attributed to an incomplete sexual education, causing poor physical and psychiatric health.

LGBTQ adolescents must negotiate the same adolescent developmental difficulties heterosexual adolescents face, with added stressors related to stigma. These additional stressors begin when LGBTQ adolescents recognize their sexual identity. Many LGBTQ adolescents endure rejection, victimization, and discrimination from parents, peers, and others, causing higher rates of psychiatric and physical problems (Human Rights Campaign, 2013). LGBTQ adolescents are more likely to attempt to lessen their heightened anguish through unproductive behavior.

Consequences of Stigmatized Status. LGBTQ adolescents are more likely to engage in unhealthy behavior to alleviate their unrelenting stress. A report by the Centers for Disease Control and Prevention (CDC) discovered that LGBTQ youth, compared to heterosexual youth, have a greater prevalence of health-risk behaviors in seven out of ten health behavior categories. These health-risk behaviors include attempts at suicide, tobacco use, alcohol and other drug abuse, risky sexual behaviors, and poor weight management (Centers for Disease Control, 2011). Although these behaviors are unproductive, they serve to ease the pain of the stressors, albeit temporarily (Burton, Marshal, Chisolm, Sucato, & Friedman, 2013).

Adolescence is a difficult development stage for most people, despite individual differences. For adolescents who represent the dominant culture, early sexual awareness can produce a mixture of excitement and confusion. However, LGBTQ adolescents also confront fears of rejection and victimization for their sexual identity.

Transgender Specific Disparities. Struggles for the transgender community exist throughout all facets of life, making these individuals most susceptible to discrimination, harassment, and violence. This discrimination is particularly prevalent in the workplace and health care system (Pizer, Sears, Mallory, & Hunter, 2012). The circumstances that nontransgender individuals take for granted are the insurmountable challenges for transgender individuals, such as applying for an identification card or using a public restroom. Currently, there are no federal laws to protect the transgender community. This year, California has become the first state to protect the rights of transgender students against discrimination and harassment, which has paved the way for similar laws in other states (Wetzstein, 2013). With such a large gap in legal protections, the transgender community faces much discrimination. Almost 30 percent of transgender individuals report harassment from police, the very people who serve to protect. Transphobia also affects the way in which transgender individuals interact in the health care domain. Many have reported that when they were sick or injured, they postponed medical care due to discrimination (28 percent) or lack of funds (48 percent) (Grant et al., 2011). A blatant paucity of transgender education for doctors and nurses forces many individuals to educate their providers on how to care for them (Grant et al.). The continuous disadvantages within the transgender community fuel the need for protective legislation and education.

Aging

> *It takes a village to raise a child.*
>
> —*African Proverb*

The problems of LGBTQ people who face old age in twenty-first-century America begin with the challenges that all seniors face. According to the 2009 U.S. Census, currently there are 39.6 million people sixty-five or older, or one in eight persons. However, these census figure estimates indicate by 2030 there will be 72.1 million, or one in 4.5 persons (Roszak, 2009). The vast increase is attributable to the Baby Boomer generation, as well as increased and better health care. The problems seniors face today include being labeled as "geezers" and "old fogies," rising health and care issues, as well as the perception they have little to contribute to the laissez-faire capitalism our country embraces (Thane, 1998).

However, these problems have not always been so. Research indicates that senior citizens were revered for their wisdom during the seventeenth and eighteenth centuries (Calasanti & Slevin, 2001). They enjoyed that status because young people were taught and expected to learn from their elders, either academically (the equivalent of home schooling) or from civil means like voting, or from vocational experiences, including job training and/or internship opportunities (Egendorf, 2002). Senior citizens comprised only 2 percent of the population, so they were given the best seats at social functions and church, and young people were taught to respect them for their longevity and accomplishments (Egendorf). Unfortunately, this public perspective toward the elderly changed by the eighteenth and nineteenth centuries. Before the Industrial Revolution, our society was referred to as "agrarian," which had the connotation our citizens were more often than not farmers and ranchers. Small businesses gave way to big business during the Industrial Revolution beginning in the mid nineteenth century and lasting through the twentieth century. The development of communications like telegraph and telephones, the advent of railroads and factories, where both voluntary and involuntary immigrants were invited or conscripted to fill various jobs, and the invention of labor-saving machines rendered aged workers less useful and thus less respected. Older people found there were fewer amenities like good seating at social and religious functions on the macro level. At the same time, less respect and consideration were given to the older generation from the younger people in their families and towns/cities on the micro level, who began viewing them as family burdens or even competition for employment and jobs. Moreover, as early as 1777, the first retirement laws were passed, the first "old age" homes were established, and terms like "codger" and "fuddy duddy" came into use (Cruikshank, 2009).

The plight of senior citizens in the twentieth and twenty-first century is much more complementary to the last century than it was in the sixteenth and seventeenth epochs. The advent of the "Information Revolution" highlighted four ever-widening divides of seniors versus their younger counterparts. The first is society fears aging, and seniors are placed "outside the box" by a culture that reveres youth and does not respect longevity (Roszak, 2009). Second twenty-first-century America has been inundated with television and media to believe that the culture of youth must be not only be observed but also revered and cultivated. Third, the 1980s' Social Security debates refocused the 1960s' "generation gap" into "the war between the generations." Last is the thought that as seniors continue to live longer and longer, their care and sustenance will have to be drawn via taxes from other tax payers, specifically the "Post Baby Boomers" (Egendorf, 2002).

To address these four issues, the United States must address several situations. To begin, it might be necessary to readdress the contradictory concept of age itself. When people sixty-five and older are denied the rights to meaningful employment, they often sink into realms of depression, alcoholism, and a combination of self-medicating drugs and/or short- and long-term illnesses. Second, when seniors do need necessary medical care, there is the chance they could be even more useful, contributing citizens. Third, many seniors tend to live by themselves, but when it does come time for them to leave their homes, they are often relegated to treatment centers, assisted living arrangements, or full-care homes. Rarely are they allowed to choose the placement and/or the types of treatments and activities they must accept. Last, placing seniors together in homes may be convenient for society, but it might also hinder the creativity and individuality that those people could offer (Berger, 1996).

Growing old in the twenty-first-century United States for senior citizens is fraught with four important challenges. The concept of retirement is the first one, and only after the Social Security Act of 1935 was the age of sixty-five marked as the conclusion of full-time employment, but it was also the beginning of their dependence on either the government, their families, and their husbands and wives (Calasanti & Slevin, 2001). As seniors face retirement, the fear of loneliness and isolation occurs, both for individuals and for their partners. Last, seniors face the fact their families and society in general often view them as a burden, for matters of inheritance and intensified emotions, and medical care is often needed. Seniors, who once provided for themselves and their families, now face having to care for themselves and their partners, often without the abilities to do so (Thane, 1998). It is said "youth is wasted on the young," but it is also true that senior citizens, who once thrived in a culture that worships youth and productivity, face severe challenges in their latter years. The irony is that the younger generation often do not respect and/or help their elders but will soon join that exclusive club.

Senior citizens who come from the LBGTQ community not only incorporate the many stigmas and problems of their heterosexual counterparts face but also add several other important problems. There are two distinct "recognition" factors that must be overcome if LGBTQ people/citizens are to complete what the media calls the "golden years" in harmony and satisfaction. The first one is that LGBTQ seniors must keep psychosocial stress from becoming the overwhelming (medical) "perfect storm" it might become from its own community (Calasanti & Slevin, 2001). That is to say, ageism within the LGBTQ community leaves individuals without the emotional support necessary to age well.

It is important that LGBTQ people act as a unified community for any subsequent progress. As LGBTQ people age, they are going to need much unification and acceptance of each other. They will need this alliance to fight for their rights as senior citizens to combat the following psychosexual stressors both as senior citizens and LGBTQ individuals: proper health care, representation in public policies, retirement benefit equality, and social acceptance (Eaklor, 2008; Spradlin, 2012).

The paragraph below, which addresses health issues for LGBTQ people in general, is a good contextual introduction for issues relating to LGBTQ seniors. The second "recognition factor" for the LGBTQ community must come from the American society itself. To this end, Senator Michael Bennett of Colorado proposed the LGBT Elder American Act of 2012 (now referred to committee action) do the following:

- Recognize LGBTQ people as a very vulnerable population;
- Establish on a permanent basis the National Resource Center on LGBTQ Aging to use online resources, and provide underserved LGBTQ people with service providers;
- Empower the Assistant Secretary of Aging to see and use data provided by the National Resource Center on LGBTQ Aging;
- Have ombudsmen collect and use data regarding discrimination of LGBTQ people; and
- Find out how available programs and grants can help the LGBTQ community.

CONCLUSION

As this chapter has pointed out, American LGBTQ lives are fraught with the pressures of growing up, maturing, and taking their rightful places as full-fledged members of society in twenty-first-century America. Nascent adolescent awareness of sexual identity represents the beginning challenges unique to LGBTQ youth. If these challenges can be negotiated adequately through support and information, later issues may be more easily addressed. However, for most LGBTQ adolescents, negative appraisals of their sexual identity can lead to higher rates of psychiatric and medical health problems that continue throughout their lives. The elderly LGBTQ community faces ageist stigma, like their heterosexual counterparts, and the stigma of being a sexual minority. These compounded stressors lead to poor health outcomes. Public policy, workplace equality, accessible nonbiased health care, and education will facilitate social change toward a positive regard for sexual minorities. These societal changes will reduce stigma-related stressors associated with health disparities.

· 7 ·

Reproductive Physicians' Treatment of Lesbian Patients in Germany and the United States

Alicia VandeVusse

$\mathcal{I}$n the past decade, the German government passed legislation permitting civil union partnerships and prohibitions on employment discrimination based on sexual orientation. The country has also experienced the rise of multiple prominent, openly gay politicians such as Guido Westerwelle and Klaus Wowereit. American public culture appears considerably less tolerant in each of these respects. However, in the realm of reproductive technologies, the situation is reversed: The American Medical Association holds that it is "not unethical" for doctors to treat lesbians and single women, whereas the guidelines of the Bundesärztekammer (BÄK, or German Medical Association) characterize artificial inseminations as prohibited (*ausgeschlossen*).

This chapter compares the regulations relating to lesbian reproduction in Germany and the United States and explores the policies and opinions of physicians of reproductive medicine regarding treatment of lesbians. Specifically, this study investigates questions about the extent to which reproductive physicians in Germany and the United States treat lesbians, the physicians' opinions on lesbian-headed and single-parent households, and the relationship between their opinions and their willingness to treat lesbians.

Because Germany and the United States are similar in their level of industrialization, economic power, and the visibility of alternative family structures, they provide a similar backdrop for examining these research questions in depth. However, because the legal regulation of the family and medicine differs considerably in the two nations, a comparison of the on-the-ground experiences of physicians of fertility medicine in both countries allows for a nuanced examination of how regulations influence their experiences, choices, and opinions.

This chapter begins with a review of relevant background information about policies, regulations, and laws that affect lesbian reproduction in Germany and the United States. First, the status of gay marriage legislation in both countries is briefly reviewed. Next, the legality of adoption by gay and lesbian couples, including laws regarding second-parent adoptions, is covered. Finally, this chapter provides a summary of the status of health insurance coverage for fertility treatments for gay and lesbian couples in both countries.

In the next section, this chapter describes how gay and lesbian reproduction is regulated by reproduction-specific laws in both countries. Germany's Embryo Protection Act has important implications for gay and lesbian reproduction, as it outlaws several treatment options that are commonplace in the United States, such as surrogacy, egg donation, and the implantation of more than three embryos. In addition, laws regarding sperm donation and the rights of sperm donors affect lesbian reproduction, as do the guidelines put forth by professional medical associations in Germany and the United States.

After establishing the regulatory context in both countries, the theoretical frameworks of stratified reproduction and medicalization are used to interpret the findings from this comparative study of the policies and practices of reproductive physicians in Germany and the United States. The data presented come from semistructured, open-ended interviews with doctors of reproductive medicine in Germany (n=15) and in the United States (n=12).

BACKGROUND

This section provides information about the legal rights and privileges granted to gay and lesbian individuals and couples in Germany and the United States, including marriage, adoption, and insurance coverage for fertility medicine. Because the legal status of each of these rights is in flux, what follows can be considered accurate as of July 2013. All interview data discussed in this chapter were collected prior to this point, and thus changes in the laws after this do not affect the responses recorded here.

Marriage Rights

Germany passed a law allowing registered partnerships (*eingetragene Lebenspartnerschaft*) throughout the country in 2001. Although these partnerships were originally distinguished in several ways from heterosexual marriage, the years since have brought about the elimination of many, though not all, of the legal distinctions. In 2004, the Life Partnership Law Revision Act expanded the rights allowed to registered partners by simplifying divorce and alimony rules and allowing some adoptions. Rulings by the Federal Constitutional Court in Germany *(Bundesgerichtshof)* have since granted registered partners broader inheritance taxation rights, adoption rights, and joint tax filing benefits.

In the United States, President Bill Clinton signed the Defense of Marriage Act (DOMA) into law in 1996. DOMA restricted federal recognition of marriage to heterosexual couples by specifying that the federal government understands marriage as between a man and a woman. Since DOMA's passage, individual states have granted varying degrees of recognition to same-sex couples, with thirteen states and the District of Columbia currently recognizing same-sex marriages and six others allowing some form of civil union or domestic partnership (Lambda Legal, 2013b). The legal rights and privileges given to these unions are complicated by the federalist form of government in the United States, as certain rights are granted at the federal level (such as immigration and forms of taxation) whereas others are administered at the state level (such as adoption rights). Even though the Supreme Court invalidated key portions of DOMA in July 2013, marriage benefits for same-sex couples remain largely confined to the limited number of states that have legalized same-sex unions.

Adoption Law

As noted above, Germany's original registered partnership law did not cover adoption law, but the 2004 revision allowed registered partners to adopt one another's biological children (i.e., second-parent adoptions or stepchild adoptions). In 2013, the Federal Constitutional Court of Germany further ruled that registered partners must be allowed to adopt one another's adopted, non-biological children. However, registered partners remain unable to jointly adopt a child. Because German law allows unmarried people to adopt, it is possible for one person in a gay or lesbian relationship to adopt a child, but not both. Although such adoptions are legal, the chances of a gay or lesbian person (or a single heterosexual person) successfully adopting a child are extremely low. Adoption agencies and birth parents often prefer for adoptive children to be placed in married, heterosexual households, and there are fewer domestically adoptable children than persons wishing to adopt. The situation is similar for international adoptions (Bundesministerium für Familie, Senioren, Frauen und Jugend, 2013). Thus, despite the relative ease with which German gay and lesbian couples won legal recognition of their partnerships, they have been unable to secure access to the full adoption rights that married, heterosexual couples enjoy.

In the United States, adoption law is regulated at the state and local level, and thus there is a haphazard array of laws regarding adoption by same-sex couples. Because local courts often determine custody, there can even be variation within a jurisdiction. Furthermore, "[a]bout half of all states permit second-parent adoptions by the unmarried partner of an existing legal parent, while in a handful of states courts have ruled these adoptions not permissible under state laws. This leaves parents in many states legally unrecognized or severely disadvantaged in court fights with ex-spouses, ex-partners or other relatives" (Lambda Legal, 2013a). In addition, many states have ambiguous or nonexistent laws regarding adoption by gay and lesbian couples, leaving many cases up to the decidedly variable discretion of the legal system.

Insurance Coverage

Access to reproductive treatment is regulated through health insurance coverage of treatments, in particular regarding the ways in which insurers limit coverage for treatment, based on personal factors such as marital status and, by extension, sexual orientation. Almost 90 percent of Germans have health insurance through the statutory insurance program, which ensures partial coverage for certain fertility treatments (Rauprich, Berns, & Vollman, 2010). For example, since 2004, the statutory health insurance covers 50 percent of the cost of three rounds of in-vitro fertilization. However, payment for these treatments is restricted to women between the ages of twenty-five and thirty-nine years old and men between twenty-five and forty-nine years old. In addition, "treatments of non-married couples or of HIV-positive patients, and treatments involving third parties, meaning any treatment involving sperm donation, are completely excluded from coverage" (Rauprich, Berns, & Vollman, p. 1226). According to the statutory health insurance plan, then, appropriate uses of reproductive technologies are defined as those that aid the heterosexual married couple in producing offspring genetically related to both parents. Lesbian couples, single women, and even unmarried heterosexual couples are expected to pay the full cost of assisted reproductive treatments themselves.

Whereas these policies apply to the entire country of Germany, each American state has different health insurance laws, and only fifteen states currently require some level of insurance coverage for fertility treatments (Arons, 2007; Resolve, 2013). In states that do require such coverage, treatments are often covered only for married couples, although this sometimes will include lesbian couples in civil unions or marriages in states where they are recognized. Thus, in both countries, insurance statutes codify appropriate users of reproductive technologies as households with two heterosexual adults who are married, although in the United States that definition is gradually expanding to include legally partnered same-sex couples as well.

Overall, regulations in Germany more clearly define appropriate users of reproductive technologies as married, heterosexual couples, whereas in the United States there is more regulatory openness regarding the appropriate clientele. The remainder of this paper discusses the study's findings regarding physicians' engagement with these visions of appropriate patients in their practices in Germany and the United States, in order to explore how the different regulatory contexts affect lesbians' access to reproductive treatments, as well as how physicians respond to the regulations on their practices.

REGULATIONS ON REPRODUCTIVE MEDICINE

Before describing into doctors' practices in these two countries, the regulatory context in which these physicians operate must be understood. Though space limits the level of detail provided here, an overview of the regulatory circumstances in Germany and the United States is presented to provide context for the results discussed in this chapter.

Legislation Regulating Assisted Reproduction in Germany

The Basic Law in Germany (*Grundgesetz*) provides constitutional protection for implanted embryos and fetuses, giving embryos "the same right to life and dignity that all persons have" (Robertson, 2004, p. 194). This is because the German Parliament responded to developments in reproductive technologies, or specifically, the ability to create embryos in the laboratory for research purposes by passing the Embryo Protection Act (*Embryonenschutzgesetz*) in 1990. This act protects certain rights of embryos, recognizing them as an early form of human life that is subject to governmental protection. Thus, the Embryo Protection Act forbids several activities that are commonplace in reproductive medicine in the United States. Specifically, one cannot transfer more than three embryos in any one cycle of in-vitro fertilization, nor can one fertilize more than three eggs at a time. In addition, egg donation and gestational surrogacy are prohibited. Each of the aforementioned activities can be prosecuted as a crime, with a maximum three-year prison sentence (Robertson, p. 205).

The passage of the Embryo Protection Act resulted from a broad political consensus, made possible by the memory of the Nazi crimes. In short, the Green Party and the Social Democrats supported the Embryo Protection Act because of their fear that reproductive technologies could be used for eugenic purposes, whereas the Christian Democratic Union supported the act based on the position that embryonic life is deserving of protection. As political scientist Nicole Richardt (2003) writes, "In sum, the specific framing of the debate in terms of continuity of life supported the demand for a comprehensive protection of the embryo. . . . Through references to historical legacies of a positive population policy, embryological research could be framed in terms of opening Pandora's box rather than making progress" (p. 110). Thus, German law takes a much stricter stance than American law with regard to reproductive technologies that involve embryos. However, because the Embryo Protection Act does not cover sperm donation and artificial insemination directly, the professional guidelines of the German Medical Association (*Bundesärztekammer*), discussed below, become all the more important in understanding the regulatory framework in Germany.

Legislation Regulating Assisted Reproduction in the United States

There is no major, binding federal regulation governing assisted reproductive technologies in the United States, and the relevant regulations exist only at the professional level. Professional regulation began in the late 1980s, with the only substantial governmental debate on the topic occurring in the early 1990s. In 1992, the federal government passed the Fertility Clinic Success Rate and Certification Act, also known as the Wyden Act, after its sponsor Representative Ron Wyden (D-Oregon). This act required that clinic-specific data on success rates for assisted reproductive technology procedures be published and that certification standards be developed for clinics handling sperm and eggs. The Centers for Disease Control (CDC) was the agency made responsible for publishing this data, beginning in 1995.

Although this activity certainly sounds like active regulation, the provisions are voluntary, meaning that a clinic that refuses to give its success rate data to the CDC faces no consequence other than being listed by the CDC as "nonreporting." Despite the lack of penalty for nonreporting, clinic compliance rates have steadily increased since the passage of the Wyden Act, with more than 93 percent of clinics reporting their results in the last published report (Centers for Disease Control, 2012). However, the data collected by the CDC cover procedures only for which both sperm and egg are used, so major methods of treatment, such as artificial insemination, are not included. In addition, there is concern that reporting success rates encourages doctors to implant more embryos than they otherwise might, as clinics wish to inflate their pregnancy rates at the expense of increasing multiple births, despite the fact that multiple births come with increased long- and short-term complications and costs.

In 2004, the President's Council on Bioethics (2011) produced a report that assessed ART regulation. The council concluded, "There is minimal direct governmental regulation of the practice of assisted reproduction," and "assisted reproductive technologies (ARTs) are regulated as the practice of medicine—with licensure, certification, professional oversight, and malpractice litigation as the chief means of regulation" (p. 174). In other words, no regulation exists that is specific to ARTs; ART treatment is regulated by the government only to the extent that medicine as a whole is regulated. Although professional self-regulation of these techniques and technologies is fairly extensive, "compliance with the standards invoked is purely voluntary" (President's Council on Bioethics, p. 175). The Council recommended various options for improving the regulatory framework, including the creation of a new federal agency to oversee ARTs (similar to the Human Fertilisation Embryology Authority in the United Kingdom), the augmentation of existing agencies, and federal legislation. However, these policy options were not pursued, and there has been little change to federal ART regulation since that time.

In the United States, the practice of medicine is primarily regulated at the state level, and thus every state has a medical board. However, many states do not have regulations specific to reproductive technologies. The state laws that do exist lack consistency and are not well developed. Furthermore, there is a huge diversity of state laws relating to ART, ranging from legislation that prohibits and even criminalizes certain reproductive options, such as surrogacy, to several states' attempts to actively encourage embryonic stem cell research. For the purposes of this chapter, the key point is that no state has enacted a comprehensive regulatory framework regarding reproductive technologies, and neither has the federal government.

Professional Regulation in Germany

In Germany, the *Bundesärztekammer* (BÄK, or German Medical Association) regulates the provision of reproductive technologies that are not otherwise covered by law. The BÄK publishes binding guidelines, and sanctions can result from failure to follow the guidelines, including loss of one's medical license. However, as others have noted, "sanctions are not very likely to be pursued" in cases where "the medical profession itself is divided" (Schmid, 2009, p. 66).

With regard to the regulation of sperm donation in the cases in which the woman is in an unmarried partnership, is with another woman, or is unpartnered, the BÄK takes a strict stance. In 2006, the guidelines published by the BÄK state that providing a child with a stable relationship to its father is of utmost importance. Thus, "for unmarried pairs, a heterologous insemination will be met with special caution; this is explained by the goal of providing the so-conceived child a stable relationship to both parental units. For this reason, the heterologous insemination is currently prohibited for women who are not in a partnership or who live in a same-gender partnership" (Bundesärztekammer, 2009). Thus, the guidelines recommend excluding lesbian partners and single women from receiving sperm donation in a medical context because the potential child would (assumedly) lack a relationship to its social and genetic father. This is in spite of the fact that anonymous sperm donation is illegal in Germany, because all donor children have the possibility to learn the identity of their donors when they turn eighteen. The overarching goal of the BÄK's guidelines regarding sperm donation, then, seems to be to guarantee that any child resulting from assisted reproductive treatments has a social and legal father.

The structure of the BÄK creates a bit of a loophole for some of this study's respondents, though, because these guidelines are issued at the national level, but each local medical association must then vote to approve the guidelines in order for them to take legal effect. Berlin's medical association did not approve the aforementioned guidelines, and thus, doctors in Berlin are not legally required to follow them. However, a related research project by this author has shown that many physicians are uncertain about this and unwilling to take what they perceive as the risk of not following their professional guidelines. One additional cause of concern for some German physicians is the controversial nature of the physician's role in conception in cases where parentage is contested. There have been rare cases where courts have held physicians financially responsible for children conceived with donor sperm when the sperm was used without adequate consent from the donor (Jüttner, 2013). These cases lead some physicians to be reluctant to treat unpartnered women, out of concern that they may be financially liable. However, such cases are rare and involve highly unusual circumstances, and their applicability to lesbian couples attempting to conceive is tenuous at best.

Professional Regulation in the United States

In both countries, professional guidelines tend to fill the void left by a lack of governmental regulation regarding artificial insemination, but professional regulation in these two countries is vastly different. In the United States, professional organizations undertake regulating functions such as accrediting clinics, sanctioning doctors who flout norms and guidelines, and reporting clinic success rates. However, professional organizations do not have the force of law behind their recommendations and guidelines in America.

In 1987, the Society for Assisted Reproductive Technology (SART) formed as an organization of professionals dedicated to the practice of ARTs in America. SART's first major undertaking was data collection and reporting of fertility clinic success rates, which it began doing voluntarily in the late 1980s. In the early 1990s, SART helped set up standards for the accreditation of ART clinics, though SART itself is not an accrediting agency. Although today the CDC is the federal agency responsible for reporting of clinic success rates (due to the passage of the Wyden Act in 1992), SART and other professional organizations still play an important role in creating guidelines for doctors regarding treatment standards.

However, being a member of SART does not necessarily mean that a clinic follows its guidelines, despite the fact that SART previously claimed to be a "governmental watchdog for ART" (Thompson, 2005, p. 229). For example, the Los Angeles, California, clinic where the "Octomom" (Nadya Doud-Suleman) underwent IVF was a member of SART prior to the octuplet birth.[1] After the scandal, the physician, Dr. Michael Kamrava, had his membership in SART rescinded, and his medical license was also revoked by the California Board of Medicine for "gross negligence." Indeed, the publicity surrounding the octuplets led to renewed calls for governmental oversight and regulation of fertility clinics, but no major legislation resulted.

The American Medical Association (AMA) publishes general guidelines regarding artificial insemination. It is in these guidelines, published online, that the AMA states, "In the case of single women or women who are in a homosexual couple, it is *not unethical* to provide artificial insemination as a reproductive option" (American Medical Association, 2004, para. 5; emphasis added). The inclusion of this sentence allows fertility doctors to treat single heterosexual women as well as lesbians without fear of professional sanctioning. The only other statement that the AMA guidelines make regarding family composition in families created with ART is: "The consent of the husband is ethically appropriate if he is to become the legal father of the resultant child from artificial insemination by anonymous donor." Thus, the AMA presumes that a heterosexual couple undergoing treatment with donor sperm is married, which could raise questions about how doctors should proceed if confronted with an unmarried heterosexual couple. However, nothing in the guidelines precludes treatment in such cases. Furthermore, the AMA guidelines state that: "Anonymous donors cannot assume the rights or responsibilities of parenthood for children born through therapeutic donor insemination, nor should they be required to assume them." This stance is echoed in many states' laws regarding donor insemination, in which sperm donors effectively strip themselves of their parental rights and responsibilities. Thus, the legal and professional regulation of assisted reproduction differs greatly between the United States and Germany. The following section explores the effects these differing regulatory structures have on fertility specialists and their treatment of lesbian patients.

METHODS

This is a qualitative study of the experiences and opinions of fertility physicians in Germany and the United States. Data were collected primarily in the cities of Berlin and Chicago. However, there are local differences in regulations, political landscapes, and norms as well, a topic addressed by interviewing a smaller sample in one additional city in each country (Munich and Milwaukee).

Respondents were solicited using repeated contacts through the mail, as well as through email and phone solicitations. Letters were sent to all of the doctors of fertility medicine located through extensive online researching of reproductive clinics in the cities of interest. The results come from semi-structured, open-ended interviews with doctors of reproductive medicine in Berlin (n=13) and Munich (n=2), and in Chicago (n=8) and Milwaukee (n=4). Interviews were conducted in English or German, according to the respondent's preference. During the interviews, respondents were asked general questions about their jobs, as well as questions about the clinics where they practice. Additional interview topics include how patients are selected and who is treated, physicians' broad opinions on family and alternative family structures, and their orientation toward their professional guidelines. All interviews were transcribed and coded using the qualitative analysis software Atlas.ti, and quotes from interviews have been translated by the author where applicable.

Of the twenty-seven respondents, fourteen are male and thirteen female. Twenty-four of the physicians interviewed are white, one is African American, and two are of Middle Eastern descent. The doctors were fairly evenly split with regard to age, with eight physicians in their thirties, eight in their forties, five in their fifties, and another five who are sixty years or above. As mentioned before, fifteen physicians in Germany were interviewed (thirteen in Berlin and two in Munich) and twelve physicians were interviewed in the United States (eight in Chicago and four in Milwaukee).

RESULTS

This chapter focuses on the portion of the interview in which doctors of fertility medicine discuss treating lesbians and single women and the instances where they describe their opinions about lesbian-headed and single-parent households. In particular, this chapter investigates the following three research questions.

1. Do doctors of fertility medicine treat lesbian patients in Germany and the United States?
2. How do these physicians feel about single-parent and lesbian-headed households?
3. To what extent do doctors' policies reflect their opinions versus their regulatory constraints?

Do Doctors of Fertility Medicine Treat Lesbian Patients in Germany and the United States?

The first research question investigated in this chapter is whether doctors of fertility medicine treat lesbian couples and single women of all orientations in Germany and the United States. The study's results indicate that there is a notable difference in the willingness of German and American fertility doctors to treat lesbians and single women. Among this study's respondents, nearly half of the doctors interviewed in Germany stated that they do not treat lesbian and/or single patients, whereas all of the respondents in the United States mentioned treating these women as standard practice.

One German doctor, a man in his forties who was particularly adamant about his clinic's refusal, stated, "In Berlin there is a large homosexual community, and because of that we receive very many inquiries, but there are other clinics that do it; we don't do it. But we're asked about it practically every week." When asked what they told these potential patients, he continued: " . . . we say: 'We don't do that, find somebody else!' I don't actively refer them to colleague so-and-so, no." Most of the doctors in Germany who refused treatment, however, espoused the idea that every patient should still be offered an advising appointment. As another male Berlin-based doctor in his fifties stated, "We might advise them, but we can't help them," going on to explain that these treatments were not condoned by the professional guidelines. Additionally, one older, male doctor references these women's social, rather than medical, infertility as precluding treatment: "These women have no medical condition, so why would I treat them?" Thus, a range of justifications underlies the policies of many fertility clinics and physicians who refuse fertility treatment to lesbian and/or single women. Regardless, these views lead to unequal access to care for lesbians and single women of all orientations seeking reproductive treatment in Germany.

By contrast, all of the doctors interviewed in the United States indicated that they treated lesbians and/or single women, as did over half of those interviewed in Germany. In both countries, these doctors often expressed the idea that it is not their job to judge who is fit to parent, particularly given that people without fertility issues (whether social or biological in nature) receive no screening before they reproduce. Their job, as they themselves frame it, is simply to do whatever they can to help people conceive. Because there are doctors who hold these beliefs and act accordingly, lesbian women are likely able to find providers willing to inseminate them, at least in large metropolitan areas in both Germany and the United States. These doctors were generally unconcerned by the professional guidelines sanctioning treatment in cases without a social father; in fact, one doctor mentioned having had no success trying to discover if anyone had been professionally sanctioned for failing to follow the BÄK's guidelines.

All of the doctors interviewed in the United States indicated that they see lesbian patients with some regularity. Most doctors estimated that the percentage of their patients who were in lesbian couples fell between 3 and 5 percent, with a similar percentage of single women coming in for treatment. Every doctor interviewed in the United States mentioned that treating lesbian couples, as well as single women of all orientations, was acceptable to them and undertaken by their clinics regularly. This contrasts sharply with the situation in Germany, where many doctors and clinics simply refuse to see patients who disclose that they are single or part of a lesbian couple. Thus, the effect of the regulatory context is highly visible in the simple difference between the number of physicians in Germany and the United States who are willing to treat lesbian and single women of all orientations.

How Do Respondents Feel about Single-Parent and Lesbian-Headed Households?

The second research question posed in this chapter explores the physician respondents' opinions regarding lesbian couples and single women parenting, as well as the importance of male and female role models for children. During the interview, physicians were asked questions about family structures with an emphasis on their personal opinions (and assurance that they would remain anonymous). In particular, participants were asked if they thought that children should have two parents and if children need to have male and female role models. Their answers to these questions reveal the complex ways in which reproductive physicians' policies regarding the treatment of lesbians and single women both uphold and contradict their own views about family structures. Indeed, inconsistencies in their personal beliefs and their practices regarding nontraditional patients were quite common. In particular, many doctors who indicated a willingness to treat lesbians and single women nonetheless asserted that it is better for children to have two, differently gendered parents. For instance, one female interviewee in her late thirties, who works at a Munich clinic where both lesbians and single women are treated, nonetheless expressed a preference for two-parent households and male role models, evidencing some self-contradictory beliefs as she spoke.

> Well, I believe that it's great, when one has two parents. By which I don't mean that one needs man and woman. So one knows very well by now from studies that even lesbian couples . . . that [their] children can grow up really well. There aren't that many gay [male] couples that have children. . . . I think it's great, that I have a father and a mother, right? But I think that there are also many mothers, who are left by their husbands and who can give a really good family atmosphere [to their children]. So I believe, that these days one has to be a bit flexible. One may not say that only *this* is a family, and all the rest is bad. Life can present so many circumstances. I believe only that you must think really well if you are ready, even if your partner leaves you, if you're single, or something, if you have the strength and the will to, so to speak, cut back on things for your child. But I believe that it's good, when there are two [parents], but there are also many children with single mothers or fathers who are raised very well.

When she was asked as a follow-up if children need a mother and father figure, she further replied: "No. So, I mean, masculine and feminine role models are important, so with lesbian couples, I think it's important that there are men in the circle of friends. But I don't think that one absolutely needs a father or that one must have a father."

The most notable differences between statements made by the German and American doctors' opinions on family structures are visible in their responses to the question of whether children need to have two parents. The German respondents were far more likely to state that children need two parents than were their American counterparts. Nine of the fifteen German respondents indicated that they thought children should have two parents, whereas only one American interviewee agreed. That said, the remaining American respondents were evenly split between believing that it is preferable for children to have two parents and indicating that children can thrive in households including those headed by single parents.

Thus, another Berlin physician, a man in his forties, when asked if he treats single patients, replied: "There are [single women], but they are only advised, not treated. . . . We have them too, lesbian couples. They do the so-called self-inseminations. That means, they are taught by us, they receive a hormone stimulation before, we do that all together and then they do the insemination themselves . . . here. And what we don't do with them is in-vitro fertilization. So when the egg cells have to be extracted, we don't do that with same-sex pairs." Although he cites the legal uncertainty regarding professional guidelines as motivating this refusal, his personal beliefs regarding family structure may make this decision easier. When asked if he thinks that children need two parents, he answers: "Yes. . . . Because I think that it's good, when a child has a fatherly person and also a motherly person. . . . So it can also be two lesbians. It's not optimal, because the man is missing, but it's better than just one person alone. The worst thing in my opinion is one person alone. It can work too, everything can work, we have enough examples of single mothers, but ideally a child needs a father and a mother." At this point, he was asked if his personal opinion influences his work, to which he responds: "Yeah [drawn out], yes, of course, it's the case that for example I do not treat single women at all. I *only* advise single women, and I don't undertake any treatments. For that reason." This doctor evidences his belief in the importance of traditional gender roles in parenting when asked to elaborate about why he believes that children need male role models:

> Well, because, look, when I now think about it . . . I was just at the Baltic Sea for four days with my family, and if [my kids] had gone alone with their mother, than they would have . . . it would have still worked, but they wanted naturally, they wanted to go fishing with me and want to do certain things with their dads that mothers don't do with them or can't do with them. And there are also differences, when their fear levels are concerned. It is simply so, that with the father one can usually do certain things, that are a bit more dangerous, and it's good that way. And on the other hand it's also good, that there's a corrective from the side of the mother. So I think, nature established it this way consciously.

Indeed, the American and German respondents demonstrated a fairly similar split in their views regarding whether children need a father figure or male role model in their lives. A plurality of respondents in the United States agreed that having male attachment figures is necessary or at least preferable, and the same was true for the German respondents. Physicians in both countries often mentioned their own families when describing their beliefs, such as the German doctor quoted above and the following quote from a Milwaukee-based male doctor: "I think that men and women are different, we are created different and we bring different things to the family. I think . . . I see it in my own family, what I bring to my daughters is a lot different than what my wife brings to my daughters. I think they benefit from both of those. So . . . yeah. So I think if you are missing part of that, it's not that you can't be perfectly fine and functional. I think it's . . . you miss out, that's the problem."

Many physicians who were interviewed in the United States expressed their opinion that having two parents was "easier" or "nicer" than having a one-parent household. However, these same physicians clearly described their belief that growing up in a variety of family situations was not necessarily harmful to children's development. Indeed, just over half of the American respondents indicated that they thought having two parents was preferable. The following quote from a Chicago-based physician represents the characteristic response of American physicians to the question of whether they think children need two parents: "No, not necessarily. I mean, it would be nice. But would it be—is that ideal? Yes. But can you have a child who's, you know, perfectly well-adjusted and happy with one parent? Yeah." Similarly, many of the physician respondents in the United States felt that having a male role model was crucial to children's development, though they were quick to specify that such a role model need not be a parental figure for the child.

To What Extent Do Doctors' Policies Reflect Their Opinions Versus Their Regulatory Constraints?

Although it is not possible to determine conclusively why more of the physician respondents in Germany refuse to treat lesbians and single women than in the United States, there were signs that both the regulations and their personal beliefs play a role in motivating these policies. For instance, one Berlin-based, male doctor in his fifties explained that his clinic refused to treat single women of all orientations because of legal restrictions, whereas lesbian couples are treated so long as the nonbirth mother plans to adopt the child after birth. This willingness to treat lesbian couples, but not single women, relates to the legal concerns that physicians have regarding sperm donation in cases without a second financially responsible adult mentioned above. Even though this doctor cites the legal situation in Germany to explain his clinic's position, his personal beliefs regarding the necessity of two parents indicate that his own views may also influence this policy:

> In general I would say yes [that children need two parents] . . . I would say, OK, normally it's easier for the children to have two persons with them, one female and one male, normally in the family. The role of females and males are different, so. . . . And in general if you look from an anthropological background, to the history of man worldwide, you can say, 'OK, in most of the cultures you have a female and a male and the children will grow up with a female and a male.' So from this psychological and anthropological background, it seems to make sense that there are two persons. . . . But that does not mean that the welfare of this child is not possible if you have a lesbian couple. Or a homosexual couple, male couple. But in general there might be some problems involved in it. So if you have children who grow up in a lesbian couple, there is always a problem that the male is not visible for the peers that they grow up with in school, so there are a lot of questions raised in that respect. That does not mean that they grow up in a psychologically unhealthy condition. But it's possible that these questions will be raised and that there might be some difficulties for the children in that respect.

Thus, this physician notes that he believes children with same-gender parents may face additional problems in life, but they will not necessarily be psychologically harmed. He goes on to elaborate that, in fact, he does not perceive his work to be influenced by his personal beliefs, and he stresses the importance of patient autonomy in determining treatment options:

> If the legal situation were better in Germany, then it is up to the patient to decide because then you can follow the patient's autonomy. From the ethical background the patient's autonomy is the, from my point of view, the most important thing. Unless it is not possible to follow the patient's autonomy. And you cannot follow the patient's autonomy if you have either legal restrictions or as I stated before restrictions regarding the welfare of the child as a psychiatric matter. But [a] patient's autonomy mainly is the most important thing, and also if I have a, some ideas that there might be some major, some minor problems, let me say, [with] lesbian couples, that is not important enough *not* to follow the patient's autonomy.

Clearly, then, some physicians in Germany find themselves unable to follow their best professional judgment regarding treatment due to the legal restrictions on their practice. Although doctors in both Germany and the United States frequently indicate that they personally believe that two parents, specifically two differently gendered parents, are preferable for child development, the vast majority of these physicians nonetheless believe that these lesbians should be treated. Among the respondents in America, even physicians who believe that two heterosexual parents provide a better home environment for children nevertheless treat lesbians and single women. It seems, then, that the legal restrictions in Germany encourage discriminatory practices, whereas physicians in the United States, lacking regulatory reasons to exclude lesbians and single women from care, tend to provide treatment for alternative family structures even when these go against their personal opinions.

DISCUSSION

Germany's regulatory situation has created a health care environment in which access to reproductive treatments is clearly stratified by sexual orientation and relationship status, with real effects for lesbian women and single women of all orientations. These women face discrimination when they approach certain clinics and physicians for fertility treatment, as they may find their treatment options limited by the clinic or they may be turned away entirely. These women may still be able to find providers open to treating them, as many German physicians undertake these treatments despite the professional guidelines. Indeed, the major gay and lesbian advocacy organization in Germany (*Lesben- und Schwulenverband in Deutschland*) can recommend providers open to treating lesbians. In another component of this research project, lesbian and single women were interviewed, and the women who did pursue treatment at fertility clinics described finding these providers as relatively easy, with an Internet search and friend recommendations providing clear ideas of where to go for treatment. Additionally, the interviews with lesbian and single women study have demonstrated that the discriminatory guidelines actually lead to lesbian and single women taking a less medicalized approach to reproduction than their U.S. counterparts, as German women are more likely to circumvent medical experts and inseminate at home.

However, the BÄK's guidelines provide a clear example of the system of stratified reproduction, in which "some categories of people are empowered to nurture and reproduce, while others are disempowered" (Ginsburg & Rapp, 1995, p. 3). By privileging the medical treatment of certain family types and prohibiting that of others, these guidelines lead to discrimination against women wishing to reproduce without male partners. What is perhaps most interesting in the comparison of doctors' views in both countries is that, by and large, their opinions on nontraditional family structures are quite similar. There are many doctors in both countries who describe lesbian-headed families as loving, nurturing environments for children, but there are also doctors in both countries who believe that heterosexual, two-parent families are ideal. Indeed, these interview data make clear that even those providers who are willing to treat lesbians and single women may well hold personal views against these family types. Although physicians in Germany have legal and professional restrictions that encourage them to turn away lesbian patients, their American counterparts have no such justification. Thus, the differential treatment of lesbians and single women in these two countries appears to result from the discriminatory legal and professional guidelines in Germany rather than from fundamentally different views on family.

LIMITATIONS

Although these findings are illuminating, it is important to remember limitations of this research project. This study involves a small sample size, and participants were volunteers who may not be representative of the entire population of fertility physicians. In addition, this research was conducted primarily in the cities of Chicago and Berlin, with a smaller subset drawn from Milwaukee and Munich. Thus, the findings may not be applicable to other areas of these countries. However, these findings provide an initial assessment of the differences in treatment options for lesbians and single women in Germany and the United States as well as indicating the need for future research. In particular, this study's results indicate that future research into fertility physicians' screening processes should be conducted to examine how personal biases influence treatment plans and willingness to accept certain patients. In addition, future research should explore the effects that these different regulatory contexts have on women attempting to conceive in Germany and the United States.

NOTE

1. The Octomom gave birth to octuplets after having twelve embryos implanted by a fertility specialist in California. She had six children prior to the octuplets.

III

SILENCING, VIOLENCE, AND OTHER FORMS OF INTIMIDATION OF LGBT PEOPLE

Limiting Transgender Health

Administrative Violence and Microaggressions in Health Care Systems

Sonny Nordmarken and Reese Kelly

$\mathcal{A}$ccess to comprehensive, quality health care impacts an individual's physical, social, and mental health status, quality of life, and life expectancy. Barriers to access and inadequate or delayed services leave health care seekers with unmet health needs and decreased life expectancy (2012 National Health Care Disparities Report, 2013). Stigmatized groups often face compromised health care access as a result of structural inequality as well as unequal interpersonal treatment in medical systems in the United States. In particular, transgender people encounter numerous, multitiered obstacles when seeking health care. As we will illustrate, the process of obtaining health care itself can be particularly harmful to many trans people. Thus, they experience greater health risks, decreased life expectancies, and fewer opportunities to obtain necessary medical care than cisgender ("cis"), or nontransgender, people.

LITERATURE REVIEW

For trans people, disparities in access to health care result from legal, administrative, and social systems and practices that maintain a cis-normative culture, which privileges and normalizes cisgender experiences. Several factors contribute to this cis-normativity. First, identity documentation, which starts with sex classification at birth, reifies a two-sex paradigm. What Kelly (2012) calls "administrative recognition" occurs when administrative systems officially recognize trans people's identities. This type of recognition is imperative for health access, as it requires administrators to record trans people's identities accurately and consistently. Because administrative systems obstruct sex reclassification on identity documents, trans individuals may lack valid identity documentation (Kelly; Namaste, 2000; Spade, 2011). This predicament renders them "impossible" (Spade), limiting their access to employment, public programs, and health care. At times when trans people do achieve administrative recognition, health care may remain inaccessible simply because it is unaffordable. As trans people face marriage and employment discrimination (and they are twice as likely to be unemployed as cis people), they are less likely to have financial resources or health insurance benefits (Flynn, 2006; Grant, Mottet, Tanis, Harrison, Herman, & Keisling, 2011). They also face overt discrimination in health benefits systems. Many health insurance companies and almost half of state-sponsored public programs in the United States explicitly exclude coverage for transition-related health care (Gehi & Arkles, 2007). Additionally, both public and private benefits systems exclude undocumented trans immigrants, leaving them to navigate immigration law enforcement, legal mandates, and community-oriented health care services that may or may not be trans-inclusive (Heyman, Nunez, & Talavera, 2009). These institutional discriminatory practices amount to administrative violence (Spade).

In addition to structural barriers to access, inequities also manifest in the quality of health care trans people receive. Markedly, trans people who are able to access medical care commonly endure derogatory, negligent, or harmful treatment. Cissexism plays an important role in this problem. Although a wide range of populations experience mistreatment by health care providers, such as those who are HIV positive, poor, sex workers, fat, or non-English speaking, to name a few, mistreatment specific to trans individuals is rooted in the cissexist notions that sex and gender are binary and immutable categories, and that trans people lack the epistemological legitimacy and authority to authenticate their own sex and gender identities (Serano, 2007). Sexing individuals without consent at birth, requiring that a medical or legal administrator validates a person's sex in the reclassification process, and interpersonally acting as the arbiters of a trans person's "real" gender render cis people legitimate and trans people illegitimate gender authenticators (Kelly, 2012). In addition, cultural tropes represented in media maintain transphobic stereotypes, characterizing sex or gender shifts as strange, unnatural, fake, or monstrous (Serano). These erroneous, dehumanizing perceptions shape health care workers' behavior and take shape in microaggressions.

Microaggressions are everyday interpersonal communications that send negative messages to individuals on account of their perceived membership in or affiliation with a marginalized group (Sue, 2010). These messages are manifestations of oppression woven into the social fabric of ordinary life (Kitzinger, 2009). Whether conscious or not, all individuals enact microaggressions, many of which are routine, unintended, and invisible to both deliverers and recipients. They are verbal, nonverbal, and environmental, appearing in a range of articulations from facial expressions, body language, terminology, remarks, and representations, to the operation of institutionalized arrangements, such as rules and policies. The term "microaggression" is somewhat of a misnomer, as such actions, when examined individually, are not necessarily small or aggressive. Nevertheless, as these actions are repetitive, and at times are delivered en masse, they have great impact. Social distancing, dismissal, invalidation of a person's experience of reality, and indirect denigrating comments are non-aggressive kinds of microaggressions. Blatant discrimination, which is not "micro," can be understood as a form of microaggression if there is a possibility that perpetrators are unaware that their actions are derogatory or hurtful.

Sue (2010) created a microaggressions typology, which includes: micro-insults, or unconscious and unintentional insulting communications; microin-validations, which invalidate experiences of reality and discrimination; and microassaults, which are blatant and conscious. Applying Sue's typology, Nadal, Skolnik, and Wong (2012) describe twelve categories of microaggressions that trans people experience, including misgendering, universalizing of trans experience, exoticization, discomfort/disapproval, endorsement of gender normativity, denial of cultural transphobia, denial of one's own transphobia, sexual pathologization, physical threat or harassment, denial of privacy, familial microaggressions, and systemic and environmental microaggressions. As Kelly (2012) reminds us, "gender expressions and [trans bodies] are highly racialized and, as such, racial, national, and ethnic identities [and their associated dehu-manizing stereotypes] become intertwined with any threat trans people pose as sex/gender 'others'" (p. 9; see also Gehi, 2009; Mogul, Ritchie, & Whitlock, 2011; Spade, 2011; Vidal-Ortiz, 2009). Thus, in addition to delivering trans-phobic, cis-normative and cissexist microaggressions, individuals may mobilize transphobia, cissexism, and cis-normativity as a basis for racist and racialized microaggressions.

Trans people commonly encounter microaggressions in a number of sites in their everyday lives, such as workplaces, religious venues, and public restrooms, and potentially from any individual they interact with, from family members to strangers (Kidd & Witten, 2008; Nadal et al., 2012). In this chapter, we expand on this discussion by examining the particular kinds of microaggressions trans people experience in health care systems. We define microaggressions as interactions that communicate "othering" messages, referencing gender nonconformity, that make transness an issue, or that cause trans people to feel self-conscious of their transness.

These often unintentional slights, snubs, or insults are embedded within a larger stream of communication. They can be confusing to receive and difficult to notice, pinpoint, or recognize, leaving them particularly challenging to address, which can amplify the stress they cause. The negative impacts of microaggressions, such as chronic health problems, post-traumatic stress, or persistent anxiety, anger, depression, fear, hypervigilance, fatigue, shame, loneliness, and/or hopelessness (Pauly, 1990; Schrock, Boyd, & Leaf, 2007), are comparable to those caused by catastrophic traumas (Sue, 2010). In addition, as a result of their experiences with and knowledge about transphobic interactions and perhaps violence, trans people often anticipate these situations, amplifying their anxiety, hypervigilance, and fear (Kidd & Witten, 2008). These experiences of subjugation accumulate, creating a form of oppression-related stress, or what Meyer (1995) calls "minority stress."

As we have described, scholars have shown what administrative violence occurs structurally, on the macro-level, and on the micro-level, in interpersonal exchanges within health care settings and elsewhere. However, we do not know what meso-level, *institutional-interpersonal processes* take place to maintain the structural systems of inequality in which transgender people find themselves. This chapter explores these questions: How does cissexist social structure manifest on the interpersonal level in health care systems? How do social actors make use of institutional processes and norms to produce and reproduce trans inequality in health care systems, and what does this inequality look like? In the following pages, we address these questions.

The purposes of this chapter are: a) to chart common and interrelated microaggressions and blatant administrative violence that trans people experience in health care systems; b) to unpack the underlying meta-communications they carry; c) to explain when and how they happen; and d) to explain how social actors use institutional processes in health care to produce inequality between trans and cis people. As we will illustrate, the ways that health care providers often interact with trans patients in the midst of treatment create inadequate and inequitable services. This analysis will demonstrate how these mistreatments are rooted in cis-normative structural forces, administrative systems, and cultural practices that set up health care workers to mistreat trans people. We attempt to contextualize the impact as it relates to and is compounded by other structural variables that determine access to care including, but not limited to race, ethnicity, socioeconomic status, education, and nationality. Furthermore, in response to negligent, disrespectful, or damaging services, trans people labor to self-advocate, discontinue care, and/or seek care elsewhere. The cumulative effect of the cis-normative systems, ideologies, and behaviors on trans health seekers is an immeasurable reduction in access to and quality of care. We recommend working toward conscientious, trans-allied health care practices that will lead to greater health equity for trans people.

METHODS

This chapter combines ethnographic research from two separate projects on trans people's lives. One project investigated trans people's experiences receiving microaggressions in everyday interactions, and the other project investigated the strategies that trans people use when negotiating different social scenarios including sex-segregated facilities and identity document checkpoints. We draw on sixty-one semistructured, in-depth, and in-person interviews to examine the particular challenges that our participants faced navigating health care systems. We chose narratives from each project that described an interaction with medical providers to supplement, lend further evidence to, and nuance the findings from the other. Because both projects focused on social interactions, structural contexts, and individual agency, there was substantial overlap in what analytical themes emerged in the data and the conceptualization of root causes that shape trans lives.

For the first project, in 2011 and 2012, Nordmarken conducted participant observations and twenty-one semistructured interviews ranging from forty minutes to three hours with trans and gender-nonconforming people in northern California. Nordmarken also conducted participant observation in the Northeastern United States, and at four LGBTQ conferences, which took place in various regions of the United States. Perhaps this study could be viewed as conservative: One might expect that research on gender non-normativity in relatively liberal, diverse places and contexts may underestimate the stigma at work in interaction. However, these sites still host cisgender norms that shape perception and inform interaction.

Nordmarken's study included people with a variety of gender identities, expressions, and experiences, such as transmasculine (female-to-male spectrum), transfeminine (male-to-female spectrum), and non- or multidirectional, such as genderqueer, gender nonconforming, or gender fluid. To get a sense of whether people who are different from each other experience similar responses to their gender nonconforming appearance (and they often do), Nordmarken interviewed people with various racial and ethnic identities, ages, education and income levels, and disabilities. However, a small sample cannot be systematically compared with experiences across populations. Nordmarken recruited five interviewees through personal networks, and fourteen through the use of social media. The strengths of snowball sampling are perhaps its limitations as well: It is effective at producing data about a specific community.

Nordmarken asked participants to describe their identity, everyday interactions in different places and contexts, instances in which their gender became an issue, and when and how they experienced recognition and misrecognition.

Nordmarken lived with an informant and interacted with others in phone conversations and digital communications, in private gatherings, and in public trans community spaces, such as political actions, religious services, LGBTQ Pride events, academic events, and art festivals—at least one hundred activities. Nordmarken wrote regular field notes and analytical memos, transcribed the audio recordings and open- and selectively coded the transcripts and the notes for themes, then analyzed the data in light of the literature.

For the second research project, Kelly conducted forty semistructured, in-depth and in-person interviews, ranging in length from seventy-five minutes to four hours, in the Northeastern United States between March and October 2009. Kelly recruited participants via online, print, and in-person communications. Although snowball sampling is the primary method of purposeful sampling when targeting nonnormative gender and sexual communities (see Mustanski, 2001; Shapiro, 2004), an online distribution of the advertisement and sampling from personal networks attracted a greater diversity of respondents with regards to age, race, disability, education, and nationality. Seventy-four individuals responded to the call for participants. Kelly chose forty that represented diversity across identity categories and compensated them $15 each for their participation; postoperative respondents were oversampled for comparative analyses. We use pseudonyms here to protect participants' confidentiality.

Kelly used a "theory-driven model of interviewing" where "the researcher's theory is the subject matter of the interview and the subject is to confirm or falsify, and above all, to refine that theory" (Pawson, 1996, p. 299). The initial questions in each interview covered demographic areas (see appendix), followed by questions that explicitly centered on the logics and strategies trans people use when negotiating their identities across four major areas: the use of identity documentation (e.g., driver's licenses and passports), the use of sex-segregated facilities (e.g., bathrooms and locker rooms), participation in gender-focused events or organizations, and in everyday life. Interviews followed a loose and repetitive script, allowing the researcher to play a more "explicit role in teaching the overall conceptual structure of investigation to the subject," and the participant "to agree, disagree and to categorize themselves in relation to the attitudinal patterns as constructed in such questions but also to refine their conceptual basis" (Pawson, p. 305). The overall effect was that participants were more actively engaged in the line of questioning and refined the project's conceptual basis. The transcripts were analyzed using a "multi-grounded theory" (Golkuhl & Cronholm, 2003) approach for themes and patterns of identity management in relation to gender identity and expression, bodily comportment, and documented identity, alongside other variables that were salient for the participant in each context such as race, ethnicity, nationality, and class.

As trans people in the cisgender-dominated world, and trans researchers in cisgender-dominated academe, we are what Patricia Hill Collins would call "outsiders within" (1986). To use Betsy Lucal's (1999) language, we have been both "socially male" and "socially female": We have been perceived and treated as male and female. However, our positions as trans researchers are from the standpoint of being both outsider as researcher and insider as trans (Dwyer & Buckle, 2009). We thus hold the status of insider-outsiders, unable to fully occupy either insider or outsider positions (Dwyer & Buckle). We have also, at times, been socially illegible and have encountered treatment in the ways those of us who embody gender nonconformity are treated. As our positionalities influence the knowledge we create (Mullings, 1999), our particular histories, contexts, and social locations shape the type of research we pursue and the data we generate: they are necessarily part of our narrative interpretation (Angrosino, 2005).

Notwithstanding, our trans statuses likely enhanced the access to participants; the comfort it may have given them may have produced "richer" data (Talbot, 1998–1999). However, interviewees who shared less in common with us may have been less inclined to reveal themselves. Although our familiarity with trans cultures and experience may enhance the depth to which we understand trans people and gendered processes, it may also limit our analysis. Certain things might seem less distinctive (Kanuha, 2000), and we may over-identify with participants (Glesne, 1999). It was important for us to, as Maykut and Morehouse (1994) suggest, acutely tune in to the activities we observed and the meanings that others made out of their experiences while also noticing how our perspectives can influence our perceptions and analyses. Nordmarken attempted, as Rose (1985) advises, to do his best to be aware of his biases, so that he could see how they shaped the data. At the same time, Nordmarken attempted to undermine the researcher-subject power dynamic and to view the process and the data as coproduced (Lloyd, Ennis, & Alkinson, 1994). Likewise, Kelly used a theory-driven interviewing approach (Pawson, 1996) to increase transparency and engage participants in coconstructing the interview.

RESULTS AND DISCUSSION

As we will illustrate, trans-specific microaggressions occur when dominant, cis-normative ways of thinking about gender and stereotypes about trans people actively manifest in social interaction. This can take shape in interactions when providers misunderstand or misinterpret trans people's identities, which invalidates the trans person's experiences of reality; when providers mispronoun or misname trans patients (using incorrect gender pronouns and their former name), inquire about their "real" identity, and deny or fail to acknowledge their gender identity, pronouns, or name; and when providers express a perception that trans people are different from cis people. Providers may display behaviors that communicate discomfort, confusion, shock, distance, awkwardness, or dismissal. These are microaggressive behaviors because they express cissexist prejudice and send othering messages. Health care providers enact trans-specific microaggressions at various times: when they are aware of the patients' trans status, when they are not, or when they perceive a patient's gender to be unusual. In addition, as these stories reveal, providers' trans-specific microaggressions often accompany medical harm or neglect. In the following pages, we demonstrate how trans people experience pathologization, sexualization, rejection, invalidation, exposure, isolation, intrusion, and coercion at the hands of their caregivers.

Pathologization and Sexualization

Medical systems define gender identity diagnoses and treatments in definitively pathologizing and sexualizing ways. The *Diagnostic and Statistical Manual of Mental Disorders* (4th ed.; DSM-4; American Psychiatric Association, 2000) classifies trans identification and gender nonconformity as mental disorders, called "Gender Identity Disorder" (GID) and "Transvestic Fetishism." Although language in the fifth edition (DSM-5; American Psychiatric Association, 2013) characterizes GID primarily by a persistent discontinuity between one's sense of self and their body, previous editions of the DSM and foundational texts on transsexual and transvestite identity development use indicators of genital dissatisfaction, desire for a heterosexual postoperative lifestyle, and the eroticization of feminine clothing to characterize trans identities and experiences (Stryker, 2008). The institutionalization of transness as a mental health disorder characterized by diagnostic criteria that sexualize trans people's desires, practices, and body parts sets providers up to deliver pathologizing and sexualizing microaggressions.

Indeed, providers do deliver microaggressions. Oberon, a white and Cherokee trans man in his mid-forties, experienced overt pathologization from his primary care physician at Kaiser. This doctor, he shared, "reacted to my informing him that I was transitioning by referring me to a psychiatrist." This action was microaggressive because it sent a message to Oberon that his gender identity made him mentally disordered. In response to the referral, Oberon complained to his doctor: "I was like, I think you think you're following standards of care, but you are really out of date and really invasive." Here Oberon referred to the World Professional Association for Transgender Health's *Standards of care for the health of transsexual, transgender, and gender non-*

conforming people (2011), which guide providers in treating trans patients. These standards were originally published in 1979 and are periodically updated to reflect current recommended best practices. Currently, it is not appropriate to refer trans people to psychiatrists to enable them to medically transition. In addition, by suggesting that a psychiatrist should be introduced into the transition process, the practitioner communicated a cissexist assumption that trans people are not able to understand or determine their gender identity on their own. This microaggression is disempowering and insulting, as it places the authority of gender identity in the realm of mental health professionals rather than the realm of individual experiences. In response, Oberon became upset, sharing, "and fuck you very much. That's just not OK with me. We had five circular conversations about this . . . I just got disgusted." He finally decided to "fire" this physician. By overtly pathologizing Oberon, this provider communicated a belief that trans people are indeed mentally disordered and appeared to be unaware that this opinion was derogatory. Regardless of his intent, the messages he sent were microaggressive.

In addition to pathologization, participants encountered sexualization. Saulo, a southern European, transmasculine person in his early twenties, encountered sexualized, body-focused scrutiny when he shared his trans identity with his first therapist at age fourteen. He recalls, "She asked if I'd be willing to have a double mastectomy and if I needed a thing in between my legs to feel like a man." These questions were intrusive, aggressive, and communicated an assumption that trans people must have surgery. As cis people often do when they encounter trans individuals, the therapist here focused on sexual body parts, dehumanizing Saulo. The way she asked these questions, especially when referring to a penis as a "thing," indicates aversion to transition-related surgeries and male bodies, which Saulo sensed and interpreted as "bullying." Coming from a therapist, whose role it is to offer support, these remarks are particularly inappropriate. Feeling uncomfortable, halfway through the session, Saulo said that he wanted to stop the therapy and leave. Her response, "You're not going to evade the problem by leaving," was unsupportive and manipulative. She failed to see what the problem was in that moment for Saulo: the negative experience he was having with her. For her, the problem seemed to be that he was trans—a pathologizing perspective, which she communicated in her approach and attitude. This therapist also disclosed to Saulo's parents private information that Saulo had confidentially told her about his sexual identity and gender, thus unethically denying his privacy and communicating that he was not important enough to deserve professional discretion.

It is in some way not surprising that Oberon and Saulo experienced these microaggressions. For more than half a century, the main guidebooks for mental health practitioners pathologized and hypersexualized trans people.

Furthermore, the process of seeking gender-confirming health care and/or sex reclassification authorizes mental health professionals and administrators to determine if and how a trans person is "real." Nevertheless, the cultural context does not excuse microaggressive behavior. It does, however, offer insights into the roots of the problems and why they manifest, despite the good intentions of individual practitioners.

Shock, Awkwardness, and Avoidance

Another pattern of trans-specific microaggressions include behaviors and messages that communicate opinions that a trans person is a freak, oddity, or impossible subject. Serano (2007) contends that the media and certain "feminisms" play a large role in maintaining these dehumanizing perceptions of trans people. In general, media sensationalize how trans people perform gender, fixating attention on trans women. Two main archetypes of trans women consistently appear in mainstream media: the "pathetic transsexual," who is not recognized as a woman, and the "deceptive transsexual," who villainously betrays people by hiding her trans status until her dramatic reveal at the climax of the story (Serano, pp. 36–37). Both are depicted as "freaks" and neither as a "real" woman. Similarly, some "feminist" representations of trans women that appeared in the late 1970s and continue to appear today characterize them as "dupes of gender," "technologies of patriarchy," and "rapists" (see Serano). Aside from the dehumanizing depictions of trans feminine people, there are even fewer portrayals of genderqueer, gender nonconforming, and trans masculine people in mainstream media. If providers have limited exposure to trans people and their bodies, their perceptions will be heavily shaped by these cultural representations of trans people as artificial, as freaks, and as less than human. Many of our interviewees experienced their medical providers as shocked, avoidant, and generally awkward. These responses are likely due to unfamiliarity with trans people or internalized transphobic ideas.

Diamond, a white trans man in his mid-thirties, had a negative experience with a nurse after his hysterectomy procedure. "She [the nurse] was really awkward. She wouldn't even look at my parts properly when she had to put in a catheter . . . She looked close enough to know where to put it, but then looked away," he said. "It felt like she was avoiding being around me . . . I could just pick up on this vibe that she didn't feel comfortable around me." In avoiding looking at or interacting with Diamond, the nurse distanced herself from him. This was microaggressive, as it communicated a denigrating message that Diamond's body disturbed her. Her avoidance prevented her from doing her job competently and brought about stress, alarm, and fear in Diamond, who was dependent on her as a caregiver. "It was really scary because I needed her full attention. At the same time, I didn't want her up in my business, but she had to be, to put in a catheter. There was no way around it." In this situation, Diamond had to overcompensate for the nurse's neglect and demand that she maintain a gaze with his genitals in order to properly place the catheter. "I had to tell her, 'You need to look at my parts,'" he recalled. Because of the way the nurse treated him, Diamond left the hospital earlier than he was supposed to, which limited him from getting all the post-operative care he needed at that facility.

Social distancing is a common experience for trans patients, and in many cases, it has great impact. Like Diamond, Eli, a light-skinned African American trans man in his early forties, saw a doctor who became shocked and distracted when he learned of Eli's trans identity. Eli had recently undergone a phalloplasty (surgical construction of a penis) outside the United States and had approached a different doctor when he needed follow-up surgery after returning to the United States. Eli characterized the doctor as initially "friendly," "engaging," and "not hurried." However, when Eli told the doctor about his phalloplasty, the doctor's demeanor, tone, and body language immediately changed. Eli's surgeon acted shocked and suddenly became curt. Eli said, "All of a sudden, his answers to my questions became monosyllabic, one-word answers. A couple seconds later, he rushes out of the room and is preparing an operating room for me to go." This dramatic affective shift from warmth to coldness sent a microaggressive message to Eli that his trans body was alarming to the surgeon. According to Eli, the doctor's shock distracted him to the point of impairing his ability to focus, resulting in a failed surgery, which negatively impacted Eli's emotional and bodily health. Stated Eli, "His attitude shifted toward me, and that affected the kind of care [he gave]. . . . He did a fucked-up job, and botched [the follow-up surgery] . . . I still have problems." Eli's experience is embedded in larger structural issues affecting trans health care. With only a handful of doctors internationally who are trained in urology and plastic surgery, and who are also trans-affirming, Eli's return to the United States left him with no choice for a surgical follow-up other than to see his HMO's doctors and endure both microaggressions and bodily harm.

Diamond's and Eli's providers treated them as repugnant freaks and less than human. Not only did the microaggressions emotionally impact each of them but they were also concurrent with medical neglect, harm, and in the case of Diamond, a lapse in care from leaving the hospital before his surgical recovery had sufficiently advanced. Larger cultural factors inform this pattern of awkwardness, shock, and avoidance. Dehumanizing representations of and sheer invisibility of trans people contribute to the attitudes, perceptions, and behaviors that practitioners bring into the health care setting.

Invalidation, Misgendering, and Exposure

A cissexist culture renders trans people unqualified to authenticate their own sex and gender identity, especially in cases where their trans status is made known (Kelly, 2012). As we mentioned, laws hold that a medical professional or administrator must authenticate a trans person's gender in order for that individual to acquire gender-confirming health care or sex reclassification in their identity documentation. Because of this legal arrangement, individuals and social systems may treat a trans person's self-identification as fake, unimportant, or fraudulent. In health care contexts where records may contain one's sex assigned at birth or a previous name, providers may address trans patients by a former name and/or inaccurate pronoun, misgendering them. Legitimating a cis person's designation of a trans person's gender over their own is a manifestation of cissexual gender entitlement (Serano, 2007). We also consider it a microaggression.

Sally, a white trans woman in her fifties, observed an instance of misgendering when she took her roommate, also a trans woman, to the hospital:

> Her doctor (who was my doctor for a while; this is one of the things that prompted me to change doctors) and almost everyone in the hospital staff referred to her as "he," kept calling Sarah by Sarah's original legal name, which, granted, it's in the medical file somewhere—but that file should have been updated ten years ago when she transitioned and had her surgery, you know, went through, did all the legal name change and everything. That all should have been changed and she should be referred to as "she"/Sarah.

Calling Sarah by her former name and "he" are microaggressions because they invalidate her gender and indicate that the providers think her identity is not real or worthy of respect, or that their interpretation of her identity is *more valid* than her own. Sarah's case illustrates how administrative health care systems and groups of health care workers alike disrespect trans patients by continuing to identify them by their old names and pronouns, even after they have reclassified their sex on identity documents and records. In addition, hospital staff authorized and validated each other's misgenderings (a group microaggression), bolstering cissexist ideas that trans identities are inauthentic. Observing and receiving this repeated insult so upset Sally that she found a different doctor. This illustrates how misgendering burdens trans people by compelling them to choose between enduring a microaggressive environment or putting in the time and effort to find a new provider.

Identity invalidations can also lead to further invalidations when patients point out misgendering mistakes, illustrating how microaggressions can be multitiered. Sally related: "I asked the doc about it once and he said, 'Oh, it's just a habit.' But he didn't take note of it and continued to call [Sarah] 'he.' And that was when I started noticing that everyone else that was dealing with her calls her 'he.' And I said something about it to Sarah, and she said, 'I asked about it a long time ago, and they can't seem to get their head wrapped around it.'" Here, when Sally and Sarah raised the issue, instead of recognizing their errors, apologizing, and correcting themselves, the health care providers dismissed the complaints and continued to misgender Sarah. This is a secondary microaggression, in addition to the original one. The initial misgendering invalidated Sarah's identity, and the secondary actions swept the first insult under the rug, ignoring and invalidating both her identity and her repeated attempts at recognition. It sent an underlying message that the health care providers did not care about or respect Sarah. Sally declared, "Some will and some won't [get it]. The ones that won't, I get my business done and go deal with somebody else. Like the doc in the hospital. Unless I get hurt right outside that hospital, I will ask to be taken elsewhere." To avoid disrespectful treatment, Sally has decided not to return to certain health care establishments where providers misgender her.

In addition to this kind of misgendering, invalidations can happen when health care providers fail to acknowledge gender identities and experiences beyond the categories of man and woman or male and female. Many trans individuals experience their gender identity as outside of this binary framework. Red, who is in their late twenties, identifies as half Thai, half white, "gender non-conforming," "trans," and "genderqueer, sort of." Red goes by the pronoun "they" rather than "he" or "she." When health care providers approach their interactions with patients from a cis-normative lens, recognizing only two genders, they invalidate the experiences of those who identify as neither man nor woman, or as a different gender entirely. Red underwent such an experience from a health care provider who regularly treated trans patients:

> There seems to be a "you're a transguy" thing. They [have] . . . this kind of expectation that I want to pass as male. Sometimes I go in to a new doctor and they assume, they use the word "transguy," but to me it feels like, "oh . . . you're in the beginning of your transition." I talked to a trans doctor and it felt like he was like, "Here's the whole thing and you become a transguy with a trans doctor at [this clinic]." . . . You arrive somewhere; he totally did a map thing: "You're driving from here to [the nearby city]." That's not how I feel about [my gender]. Or like, [saying] "I've talked to other transguys" feels like homogenization of what [transguy] is.

For Red, who does not identify as a transguy, being pigeonholed into the category feels invalidating. The provider is using words and metaphors that depict a unilateral or trajectory transition model, which does not resonate with Red's experience or their health care needs. The health care providers place their conception of a "transguy" onto Red and dismiss Red's conceptualization of their own body, identity, and experience. Further, the providers attempted to channel Red into a monolithic one-size-fits-all transition route. This kind of routing takes shape in hormone prescription conventions. Red relates: "At [the clinic] someone called me, and they were like, 'your [testosterone] levels are too low, so we recommend that you should up your dose.'" Upping the dose would make Red's body appear more male, which they had previously communicated to the clinic providers that they do not want. By recommending a dosage increase, the providers appear to either not understand or to actively ignore Red's identity. Although this routing may be validating to some transmasculine people, for Red it is microaggressive because it invalidates their identity and experience of reality. Paradoxically, in a setting designed for Red to acquire gender-confirming health care, providers ignore Red's gender and harm their wellbeing. Binary ways of understanding gender and narrow, prescriptive ways of diagnosing and treating "GID" thus constrain Red's doctors' abilities to treat them appropriately both medically and interactively.

Misgendering also exposes trans patients' private information and puts them at risk of further microaggressions or victimization from others. Jack, a white trans male in his early twenties, claimed that one of the last times he went to his university's health center he "freaked out" at some of the staff because they kept calling him by his former name, Jackie: "It was awkward for me with everyone in the waiting room, having a person call me [by my birth name] . . . so I'll be having a conversation . . . then it's like, 'All right Jackie?' And [the other patients are] just like, 'Who?' . . . it felt like . . . *unwelcomed exposure*" [emphasis added]. The public exposure of Jack's birth name in this context was a microaggression that sent a meta-communication that his privacy was not important and that his self-identification was not valid enough to use when addressing him. This microaggression was both systemic and interpersonal, as neither the administrative health care system nor the health care worker accurately accounted for his gender identity. This misgendering also increased the possibility that others might call his gender identity into question or invalidate it. Jack said that he felt "pissed off" for being put in a position where he had to manage a social interaction around his identity, which he did not want to discuss with casual acquaintances. As Jack laments, these experiences of exposure often lead others to inquire about his identity and ask him to account for the discontinuities between his documented gender and presentation of self. These kinds of intrusive questions are additional microaggressions, communicating that Jack's privacy is not important and that he must explain his gender identity to cis people.

Invalidation, misgendering, and exposure are microaggressions that stem from legal, medical, and social systems, policies, and practices that delegate cis people (especially staff and administrators) and not trans people as identity authorities. Despite acts of self- and community-advocacy, we see from Sally, Sarah, Red, and Jack how microaggressions impact trans people, often to the extent that they turn away from health care systems. Leaving health care systems in the midst of treatment or altogether negatively impacts trans people's health and limits their access to care.

Intrusion, Coercion, and Isolation

Trans people face a particular kind of coercion and violence in mental health care institutional contexts. In the context of a culture that imagines trans people to be unreal, fake, pathological, and deceptive, mental health care settings can be a particularly dangerous place for trans people. The "deceptive" stereotype manifests substantial impacts when it brings about preemptive and reactive behavior in mental health care workers. This stereotype translates to inaccurate perceptions that trans people are "being manipulative" to "get what they want" (e.g., to get gender-confirming care) and problematic responses, like the idea that mental health care providers should punish trans people for this "behavior." This approach invalidates trans individuals' realities and disciplines them for (healthily) being true to themselves. Similarly, providers can perceive self-advocacy as insubordination, which can lead them to abuse trans clients under the guise of "correcting bad behavior." As we illustrate, rather than trans patients' behavior, the cis-normative, cissexist administrative health care system is the true problem.

Marie, a white trans woman in her forties, encountered misgendering in a hospital's psychiatric ward. When Marie arrived at the hospital, the nurses asked what name she would like to be called but continued to address her by her former (man's) name and "he" and placed her in a gender-segregated room with a man. By asking what name she preferred, the nurses indicated that they were aware of appropriate ways to treat trans patients with respect. Then, they knowingly disrespected Marie, using her old name and pronouns, and placed her in a room with a man, invalidating and dismissing her. These actions sent a meta-communication of disapproval of her transness and also exposed her trans identity to other patients and providers, which denied her right to privacy and increased her vulnerability to further trans-specific targeting.

In addition, in the context of a psychiatric facility, as Marie explains, there are potential consequences for correcting misgendering: "Anything you

do is interpreted as a sign of psychosis of some sort. . . . When they're calling me the wrong name, if I correct them, they might toss me in the room
and strap me down and shoot me up with Ativan. So is it worth it to make a
confrontation? Do I have the mental energy to deal with it? I didn't, so I let it
go. It really bothered me the whole time I was there." This procedure is designed to be coercive. Marie faces great *administratively mandated* risks (physical
restraint and forced drugging) if she corrects misgendering and reminds others
how to address her. To understate the problem, this scenario is insufficient in
terms of mental health care. It actually exacerbates Marie's stress and limits her
access to either internal or external emotional health resources. Marie is afraid
of the consequences, so she opts to forgo advocating for herself. She cannot
access adequate health care because she faces microaggressions and discipline
as medical institutionalizations of cisgender normativity.

　　Administrative inadequacies in health care manifest in many other ways as
well. Myke, a white trans man in his early thirties, supported by disability, had
spent time in detox and chemical dependency rehabilitation facilities prior to
as well as throughout his transition. Whenever Myke was hospitalized or entered a treatment center, health care workers placed him in a single room and
denied him the opportunity to share a room with other men. Myke identified
as "male, but not completely," had taken testosterone for over a year, and had
undergone chest surgery but had not changed the sex marker on his identity
documents or records to "M." Though he appeared male, as his medical records listed him as "female," staff refused to allow Myke to room with men
or women, thus segregating Myke from all other patients. In one instance of
an overcrowded facility, providers housed Myke in the "quiet room," which
they usually used to isolate "unruly" patients. They did not place Myke in
this room at other patients' requests but to meet administrative demands and
protocol for sex segregation. Administrators may have feared that the facility
would be liable if a cis male roommate assaulted or harassed Myke. However,
this reasoning prioritizes the welfare of the institution or facility over the safety
and wellbeing of patients. Isolating Myke was an administratively coordinated
microaggression, which sent a message to him that he did not belong and that
his presence alone was equivalent to a behavioral problem.

　　The circumstance discussed above was not Myke's only experience with
exclusionary treatment by medical personnel. Another time, hospital staff sent
Myke to a detox and rehabilitation center where the ward had been split into
a women's side and a men's side in response to increased incidences of male
patients harassing female patients. Upon noting the incongruence between
Myke's appearance and medical records, the staff refused to house Myke in
this facility. He describes:

> They look at my name and then they look at me and they look at the chart and they're like, "We're confused, I thought you were a girl." And I'm like, "Well, I have girl parts but I'm a guy . . . so, put me on the men's side." And they're like, "Well, we can't do that because you have a vagina." . . . "You're going to put me on the women's side?" And they're like, "Well, I don't know yet." . . . The room was split down the middle by a piece of tape and they put me in a chair with the tape in the middle so I was literally on both sides and they had me wait there for an hour.

This action invalidated Myke's gender identity, made him a spectacle, publicly humiliated him, and sent a message that he was a problem. In fact, the gender-segregated, cis-normative system was the problem, as it was not adequately designed to provide care for trans patients and thus resulted in misgendering and marginalization. After the hour wait, they transferred Myke to a different facility and placed him in a single room with a private bathroom and shower.

During a different experience in a rehab facility, staff members were aware of Myke's trans status and again housed him in a single room, isolating him for a third time. The night staff locked the only single unit bathroom on the ward, told Myke that he had to use the women's bathroom, and threatened to physically restrain Myke if he tried to use the men's. These actions deliberately intimidated Myke and communicated deeper messages that he was unimportant and did not deserve access to an appropriate, safe bathroom. They also knowingly and deliberately invalidated his gender identity and cornered him into a no-win situation. Myke refused to use the women's bathroom: "Women in a hospital should not have men in their bathroom. Any man, trans or [not]. . . . They're going through traumatic experiences and . . . it's not fair to them to have a man in their bathroom. . . . I was not willing to put women in that situation. . . . And the men didn't care that I was in their bathroom. . . .So, I used the men's room anyway and I did get restrained." Essentially, hospital staff physically abused Myke for his gender subversion. In each of these experiences, Myke actively declined using women's facilities in order to meet what he perceived female patients needed and to affirm his "male . . . leaning" identity. When Myke was asked whether he reported this abuse to hospital administrators, he said: "Well, I tried, let's put it that way . . . it's complicated. I got punched by a nurse just for staring at them, and I punched him back . . . and I got nearly beaten to death. . . . And like, they put a towel over my face and kind of suffocated me and it was bad. So, I, I don't bring it up." In this setting, where he is dependent on hospital staff for his well-being, Myke encountered institutionalized physical and emotional abuse (what providers called "restraining" him) for being and behaving as himself, and further abuse when he nonverbally expressed discontent and when he physically defended himself. Though these actions are overtly violent, they are also microaggressions because it is likely that the perpetrators do not see injustice in their actions. "I was mad because I'd been lied to and then treated like a weird thing that had to be put on a line," said Myke. After experiencing physical "restraint," isolation in single rooms, and the denigration of being placed on the line that separated a sex-segregated ward, Myke avoided hospitalization: "I haven't been in the hospital in about a year, which is the longest it's been for a long time. But I've realized . . . if I can figure out any other way to get through something, it's better than having to deal with that again." Though this demonstrates resourcefulness, avoiding health care systems limits Myke's access to care. Ultimately, cis-normative administrative procedures, structural forces, and interpersonal treatment combine in the medical space to downgrade Myke as a trans individual.

These microaggressions isolate, intrude on, and coerce trans people. They are the result of mutually reinforcing systems and ideologies that perpetuate inequities of authority and autonomy. Depending on health care systems that pathologize, punish, and invalidate them negatively impacts Marie and Myke. They are subjects of and subject to models of classification and care that render them vulnerable to maltreatment. Myke and Marie are further limited by their unemployment to seek out alternative facilities, practitioners, or approaches to treatment. For Myke, leaving the health care system could mean death as a result of drug addiction.

In sum, health care practitioners are paradoxically doing damage to the patients they treat. Providers treat trans people as pathological and sexualize their bodies. They behave awkwardly in the presence of trans people, if not outright avoiding interacting with trans people altogether. Health care practitioners expose and misgender trans people and invalidate their identities. They also coerce, intrude upon, and isolate trans patients. These microaggressions result in medical harm and neglect. To get through these situations, trans people either advocate for themselves, complain to higher-ups, attempt to educate their providers or find new ones, or contain their feelings. Some leave in the midst of treatment, perhaps never returning to the health care system again. Consequently, trans people experience fewer opportunities to obtain necessary medical care than cis people and institutionalized barriers to care within cis-normative health care systems, which exacerbate their health risks. The microaggressive interactions that health care practitioners have with trans patients are a contributing factor to this social phenomenon. As we have discussed, microaggressions are part of the larger structural problem of unequal access to healthcare. They occur in social contexts shaped by race, employment status, income, mental health status, and education. These factors also influence the possibility that self-advocacy will lead to respectful treatment. It is only by addressing the interrelation of each of these issues that change can be made.

RECOMMENDATIONS FOR TRANS-ALLIED HEALTH CARE PRACTICE

What might health care administrators and practitioners do to improve trans people's access to adequate health care? The microaggressions trans people encounter are repetitive, prompt painful feelings, and accumulate in minority stress. As one interviewee, Eli, noted, these interactions have "a cumulative effect." He continued, "Surgeons don't want to help you when you tell them who you are. Sometimes I feel I can do it, sometimes I'm tired of it. I do it all the time in life. I'm a patient in the hospital just trying to get through it." Eli speaks here to the position he is often in of interacting with those who are unfamiliar with trans people. He feels exhausted from needing to educate others about his life. This necessity to educate providers is an unavoidable form of unpaid labor, and as most providers are unfamiliar with trans individuals, trans patients can expect to do this labor every time they go to the doctor. Repetitively having to explain oneself and deal with others' reactions creates a form of minority stress specific to the trans experience. So, health care practitioners should not rely on trans patients to be their educators. This is, in effect, another microaggression.

The problems that we have illustrated here stem from cis-normativity and cissexism as they manifest systemically and interpersonally. Like other forms of discrimination, microaggressions are informed and shaped by societal practices and cultural expectations. They are systemic, which means that irrespective of individual prejudice, people will still deliver them unless changes are made on a larger scale. Our cissexist culture defines sex and gender as binary and immutable, renders trans people monstrous, pathological, fake, and unable to authenticate their own sex and gender identities, and authorizes cis people to determine trans people's "real" genders. When these assumptions translate into behaviors, health care providers mistreat trans patients sending blatantly hostile messages and microaggressions, and thus negatively impacting their patients' health. In response to these mistreatments, some trans people leave providers or health care systems after or even during treatment. While some seek out other providers, others opt out of the formal health care system entirely. Our recommendations for better care come from acknowledging these components. Below we outline some concrete ways providers can address the root causes of trans-specific microaggressions and work to develop more supportive health care practices.

1. Respect and Integrate Trans People's Identities

Trans people have been creating alternative ways to code gender, which depend neither on the sex assigned to them at birth, nor on an administrator's validation, but on their own internal sense of self. As Cromwell (1999) and Hale (1997) found, trans people recode and resignify bodies, so that intersubjective recognition can take place without bodily alterations. As recognition does not start and stop at the body, trans people have been creating ways to recognize each other. In many cases, they verbally communicate how they would like to be read and addressed, specifying their name and pronouns, and at times, they communicate how they identify their gender (Nordmarken, 2013).

Health care workers can follow their trans patients' lead, by authorizing them as legitimate knowers of their own identities and treating them as authorities and experts of their own experience. Providers can ask about and note their patients' stated names and pronouns and can address and treat them accordingly. In sex-segregated facilities, this might mean housing them with individuals of their identified gender, rather than with individuals of their assigned sex at birth.

Sex-segregation fundamentally creates problems for trans patients. Ideally, facilities should not sex-segregate their patients, but if segregation is necessary, they should offer trans patients the option of a separate location, ask trans patients where they would like to be and place them there. Despite popular notions, trans people are often welcomed by their cis peers into sex-segregated facilities, and their subsequent removal or exclusion may be driven by administrative mandate, not community demand (Kelly, 2012). As isolation has many negative psychological effects, providers should isolate a trans patient in a non-standard room only if the patient chooses it; they should never isolate a patient by force.

Making efforts to validate trans patients' identities may help avoid exposing their trans status and enacting other microaggressive behavior and may protect them from further targeting or discrimination. Administrators and policy makers can change procedures to facilitate administrative recognition, to streamline gender transitions (whatever their form), and to accommodate and validate trans self-definition and self-authentication. This might require thinking creatively in a nonbinary way about: how to revise intake and other forms and documents in order to record a variety of pronouns, gender identifications and the possibility for multiple changes in identification; how to include trans people in support services and institutions; and how to provide resources and benefits to trans people, which they would otherwise be excluded from or refused on account of their gender illegibility.

2. Reflect On and Change One's Own Interpersonal Practices

In order to combat the cissexist ideologies and perceptions deeply embedded in contemporary American culture, it is critical to acknowledge our internalized prejudices and assumptions about trans people and become aware of the ways these manifest in our own interpersonal interactions. Beginning from the assumption that we all have internalized negative stereotypes and perceptions of trans people will aid in building awareness of how microaggressions manifest and decrease associated ignorance and possibly shame or resistance to change. Curiosity, constant vigilance, continuous observation, and reflection on our behavior will help us notice when we enact microaggressions. When health care providers recognize their active enactments of microaggressions, they will be able to question their own latent prejudices. Only then will they be able to interrupt their behavior and decide to pursue a different route of action.

3. Approach Care Provision with Sensitivity and as a Collaborative Effort with Patients

As it is likely that trans and gender nonconforming patients have had negative and possibly traumatic experiences in health care, they may be nervous or anticipate discomfort in any sort of encounter with providers. Providers who signal their awareness of these issues and their desire to make the experience a positive and healing one indicate that they care about their trans patients, which can help alleviate patient anxiety. Treating transness or bodily difference as a nonissue and working to not show or feel shock (even if providers react inside) is a good way to help trans patients feel seen as complete human beings and not as freaks in these vulnerable situations. Familiarizing oneself with trans people and culture, such as watching films made by trans people or reading books written by trans people, can help providers to understand and normalize transness for themselves, which can also help to allay their concern about interacting with trans patients. In addition, approaching health care practice creatively, with extra care, and as a collaborative effort will help make the experience better for patients. For example, asking permission to touch a patient's body, asking patients what terms they prefer to use for gendered and sexual body parts and using those terms, inviting patients to communicate if they feel uncomfortable, or inviting them to physically position themselves in ways that feel more comfortable to them can help put patients at ease and stay mentally and emotionally present. Inviting communication and negotiation recognizes patients as experts of their own embodied experience and encourages patients to take active responsibility for their own health. If providers must do certain things in ways that patients do not prefer, providers can explain the reasons clearly and can communicate that they are keeping patients' best interests in mind.

4. Prioritize Trans Competency Trainings and Continuous Gender Diversity Education

As a majority of health care workers are unprepared to provide adequate care to trans patients, we need to make information about trans issues available to individuals working in the health care field and to prioritize this as a pressing competency issue. Because microaggressions are the active manifestation of unconscious prejudice and internalized stereotypes, some derogatory treatment might be avoided by introducing workers to information about trans people developed from trans-affirmative and advocacy-centered perspectives. Health care workers can organize and attend cultural competency trainings, trans speakers' bureau presentations, or educational film screenings in their workplaces. Introducing providers to information about providers' discrimination against trans people through the lens of microaggressions can be particularly useful, as it frames the issue as one of unawareness and makes visible the reality that all social actors deliver microaggressions. This may avoid shaming well-meaning microaggressors and may help them stay open to noticing, reflecting on, and changing their behavior.

Although professional development sessions are useful, they do not sufficiently engender trans competency. One or two trainings will probably not develop in providers an understanding of or familiarity with trans people, which, as we have demonstrated is likely to result in continued mistreatment, even when providers have the best intentions, and often even when they have expert knowledge. Some health care providers who have worked longer in the field likely received information about trans people during eras of heightened trans pathologization and may carry negative and harmful perceptions into their current practice. Therefore, what health care workers need to do is commit to ongoing education and exploration in order to familiarize themselves with trans people, develop an understanding of gender diversity and the multiplicity of gender identities, and identify the way that cis-normative sex and gender categories and expectations have shaped their own lives and how cissexism has shaped their perspectives on trans people.

5. Work Together to Change Workplace Culture

As teams of workers as well as individual providers collaboratively deliver and uphold microaggressive actions, colleagues can help each other understand microaggressions and administrative violence. They can model respectful treatment of trans patients; they can use patients' correct pronouns, gender identities, and names consistently in discussions and remind each other when they slip up; and they can offer information on trans people and the issues of inequality and injustice they face. Providers who are more aware can make affirming statements about their trans and gender nonconforming patients in front of other providers so they see that patients are not freaks or curiosities but real people they care about. They can work together to create better ways of administratively and interactively treating trans patients. Finally, they can create a shared language about microaggressions in the workplace to open up space to discuss the role oppression plays in health care provision and how they, as a community, might do things differently.

6. Develop Allyship Practices

In addition to acknowledging trans people's identities, increasing awareness about microaggressions, and changing how they perceive and treat trans people, it is similarly important for health care providers to acknowledge their role in the hierarchy of identity validation. Often referred to as "gatekeeper," health care professionals are positioned as the arbiters of authenticating a trans person's identity and procuring access to gender confirming health care and a legal sex reclassification. Providers need to question their own authority in this role and think creatively about how they might rearrange how they approach their work in order to recognize trans individuals' epistemic authority. Until we dismantle this hierarchy of identity authorization, health care professionals can use their privilege to honor trans patients' needs and advocate on their behalf.

7. Suggest and Create Policy Changes

Recognizing and changing microaggressive health care spaces are imperative to cultural change, but they do little to work against larger structural problems. Policy changes have more weight to do that. Health care providers and administrators can get involved in making changes where they have influence and beyond. Administrators in public and private health care milieu can make sure internal policies support trans patients. Specifically, health insurance companies can change their policies to cover transition-related health care. As Spade (2011) suggests, alleviating medical changes required for legal gender change would make transition much more accessible. This would also help trans people access medical care, because they could more easily obtain accurate identity documents. Developing creative ways to signify pronouns, sexed characteristics, and genders on identity documents is one idea for how to resolve the problem of the current limited, binary "M–F" requirement, which makes invisible the multiplicity and complexities of trans people's bodies and identities. To transform larger structural problems, ramping up the welfare state, socializing health care, developing social programs for trans individuals, and dismantling prison and detention systems would improve trans people's physical and emotional health.

For further resources and guides on policy recommendations, see:

National Center for Transgender Equality: http://transequality.org/
Human Rights Campaign: http://www.hrc.org/resources/entry/transgender-inclusive-benefits-for-employees-and-dependents

Women's Health, Health Care Service Utilization, and Experience of Intimate Partner Violence in the United States

Bethany M. Coston

$\mathcal{V}$iolence is a not a new social phenomena. The incidence of "stranger crime," issues surrounding violent jobs, the general violence of men's hobbies and/or sport, and acts of self-mutilation and suicide have been well documented by social scientists (Hearn, 1996, 1998; Kaufman, 1987; Messner & Sabo, 1994; Stanko, 1994). War, colonialism, terrorism, and other acts of collective and/or political violence are now often the foci for sociologists, anthropologists, and political economists.

Yet, intimate partner violence (IPV) was not considered a serious social issue in the United States until the late 1900s. In the years between the 1990 and 2000, courts all over the United States began to repeal old laws and enact new ones to protect those who are abused by an intimate partner. For instance, forty-eight states enacted or revamped injunctions that enabled courts to refrain men from abusing, harassing, and assaulting the women with whom they live, and in twenty-three states, police officers were able to arrest on "probable cause" in cases of simple or minor assault within the home, with a few states and cities going further by imposing a mandatory duty to arrest the violent offender (Dobash, 1992). During this time, date rape came into public awareness, stalking became a serious crime in most states, and a history of marital violence is considered in child custody cases and in eligibility for gun licensing and possession in some states (Epstein, 1999; Grace & Britain, 1995; Sherman, Smith, Schmidt, & Rogan, 1992; Sproul, LaVally, & Research, 1997). Then, in 1994, the Violence Against Women Act (VAWA) was passed as a part of the Violent Crime Control and Law Enforcement Act to help overburdened states deal with the issue of *domestic* violence.[1]

However, the study of violence in same-sex intimate relationships or among those who identify as lesbian, gay, bisexual, and transgender (LGBT) has been scarce. One explanation for this lies in the main theories academics and researchers use when studying violence between intimates. Specifically, feminist theories, which explain man-to-woman IPV in heterosexual relationships as caused by patriarchy: the social system in which the male gender role as the primary authority figure is central to social organization (Yllö, 1993). Taken this way, patriarchy is an incredibly inadequate and limiting explanation for same-sex IPV, when gendered power is, theoretically, more equal or not relevant in the same ways (Coston, 2011).

Sampling has also led to disparate results. Most have relied on small, nonprobability samples, and as such found that 42 to 79 percent of men and 25 to 50 percent of women who identify as lesbian, gay, bisexual, and/or transgender (LGBT), and/or men and women who report violence by a same-sex partner, have experienced some form of IPV in their lifetime (Burke, Jordan, & Owen, 2002; McClennen, Summers, & Vaughan, 2002).[2]

For those studies that use representative, probability samples, researchers typically find that both men and women in same-sex relationships and men and women who personally identify as LGBT experience a higher prevalence of IPV than men and women in opposite-sex relationships or who identify as heterosexual (Blosnich & Bossarte, 2009; Goldberg & Meyer, 2013; Greenwood et al., 2002; Messinger, 2011; Zahnd, Grant, Aydin, Chia, & Padilla-Frausto, 2010).

There is a continued need for research on same-sex IPV. Indeed, although the specific health consequences of IPV for women abused by men have been discussed extensively within the literature (Breiding, Black, & Ryan, 2008; Campbell, 2002; Coker et al., 2002; Ellsberg, Jansen, Heise, Watts, & Garcia-Moreno, 2008; Gandhi et al., 2010; Heise, 1994; Huang, Yang, & Omaye, 2011; Peckover, 2003; Ramsay, Richardson, Carter, Davidson, & Feder, 2002; Richardson et al., 2002; Wingood, DiClemente, & Raj, 2000), it has only been in the last two or three years that the physical and mental health outcomes of IPV for those abused by same-sex partners have begun to emerge (Klostermann, Kelley, Milletich, & Mignone, 2011; Lehavot, Walters, & Simoni, 2010).

What we do know is that victims of physical and sexual IPV suffer higher levels of both acute and chronic physical health problems than those who are not abused (Campbell & Wasco, 2005; Coker et al., 2002; Fischbach & Herbert, 1997; Plichta, 2004; Porcerelli et al., 2003; Wolkenstein & Sterman, 1998). Among these negative health outcomes are increased mortality, injury and disability, problems with general health, chronic pain, obesity, substance abuse, reproductive disorders, sexually transmitted diseases, vaginal bleeding, and poorer pregnancy outcomes (Campbell, 2002; Huang, Yang, & Omaye, 2011; Kovach, 2004; McCauley et al., 1995; McFarlane et al., 2005; Plichta,

2004). Women physically and sexually abused by men are likely to sustain acute injuries to the head, face, neck, breasts, or abdomen, which can lead to chronic conditions such as headaches, migraine, and constant pain (Campbell, 2002; Kovach, 2004). In terms of psychological health and emotional well-being, outcomes include, but are not limited to, depression and post-traumatic stress disorder (PTSD) (Campbell, 2002; Coker et al., 2002; Dienemann et al., 2000; Dutton et al., 2006; Houry, Kaslow, & Thompson, 2005; Jones, Hughes, & Unterstaller, 2001; Stein & Kennedy, 2001).

These health outcomes lead to women abused by men constituting a significant proportion of female patients seeking emergency medical services, obstetric care, and primary medical care (Abbott, Johnson, Koziol-McLain, & Lowenstein, 1995; Koziol-McLain et al., 2004). In quantifiable terms, for abused women, this equates to approximately $8.3 billion a year for medical care, mental health services, and lost time from work due to injury and death (Max, Rice, Finkelstein, Bardwell, & Leadbetter, 2004). Although half of the women abused by men intimates report a physical injury, only around four in ten of these women seek medical health assistance (Rennison & Welchans, 2003).

For women abused by women, the health-related outcomes of violence have not been well documented. Even though the California Health Interview Survey (2007 and 2009) and the Centers for Disease Control and Prevention's (CDC) National Intimate Partner and Sexual Violence Survey (NISVS 2013) released detailed reports on same-sex victimization, this data has yet to be used to examine health disparities related to violence in relationships.

Additionally, "the short and long-term effects of domestic violence are health care issues that nearly every practicing physician encounters in the course of routine clinical practice" (Alpert, 1995), but no study using a representative, probability sample has assessed whether or not there are disparities in negative health outcomes and/or disparities in health care/medical service utilization between women abused by women and women abused by men after an experience of violence; i.e., given the similar to higher rates of intimate violence, do women abused by women suffer injury at the same rate, and if they do, are those abused by a same-sex partner seeking out medical and psychological care services just as often than those abused by an opposite-sex partner?

This analysis examines these very issues: First, by examining types of violence experienced between same-sex partners compared to opposite-sex partners, noting not just prevalence rates but also significant differences; then, by comparing negative health outcomes (physical and psychological) of said violence; and finally, by examining the medical and psychological health care-seeking and utilization behaviors, controlling for injuries suffered.

FRAMEWORK

As the topic of health outcomes and health-care-seeking behaviors of women abused by women has been understudied and undertheorized, this project is aimed at grounded theory. In general, female victims of IPV are less likely to receive needed medical services and more likely to have a poor relationship with their health care provider (Plichta, 2007). This stems mostly from the health care system's inconsistent response to IPV; most health care systems are not equipped to assist either victims or the providers seeking to help victims (Fugate, Landis, Riordan, Naureckas, & Engel, 2005).

Previous qualitative studies confirm that in addition to the health care system itself, social, political, and cultural barriers also keep victims of same-sex IPV from seeking help, which leads to the "double closet"—feeling the need to keep secret not only one's sexual orientation or intimate relationships but also the abuse and trauma they are experiencing (McClennen, 2005; St. Pierre & Senn, 2010).

Findings from discussions with advocates and health care professionals in New York City showed that the health care environment is heterosexist[3] and gender-normative.[4] Providers lack knowledge about health disparities affecting LGBT people. LGBT individuals experience hostility and discrimination in care, and concerns about homophobia and transphobia keep LGBT individuals from using health care services (Grant et al., 2010).

This lack of training and "cultural competence" may also cause care providers to misdiagnose or underestimate the extent of emerging disorders in the LGBT population (Ida, 2007; Logie, Bridge, & Bridge, 2007). Poorly trained medical practitioners may even make the mistake of viewing homosexuality and gender nonconformity as illnesses that can be overcome with appropriate "reparative" therapy, further amplifying the trauma that these men and women experience every day because of perceived LGBT status (Dean et al., 2000; Haas et al., 2010).

The social stigma surrounding "alternate" sexualities and relationships (Poorman, Seelau, & Seelau, 2003) also produces several large structural problems that prevent the primary care system from being able to adequately meet the mental health needs of LGBT youth and adults. These include: lack of LGBT-specific training for health care providers (in schooling or mandatory employee workshops), lack of financial incentives to treat LGBT youth (who may not have health insurance or do not want to use their parent's), a failure to deal with the intersection between mental health and substance abuse issues, and a general lack of information about LGBT health needs (Eliason, Dibble, Gordon, & Soliz, 2012; Winter, 2012).

Analytical Propositions

Given this framework and the previous research on IPV and health, the following outcomes were hypothesized:

1. IPV is more prevalent in same-sex partnerships than opposite-sex partnerships.
2. The negative health outcomes of IPV affect all people, regardless of the sex/gender of the survivor or abuser.
3. Those who experience same-sex IPV seek out and use physical and mental health care services less often than those who experience opposite-sex IPV.

Design

Data come from the "Violence and Threats of Violence Against Men and Women in the United States, 1994–1996" subsection of the National Violence Against Women (NVAW) Survey, a telephone survey of men's and women's experiences with violent victimization. The National Violence Against Women Survey measures the most forms of violence, includes a question to categorize sexual orientation, and is commonly used today by researchers. Although dated, it is the best available dataset on forms of LGB and/or same-sex violence.

The national sample was drawn by random-digit dialing from households with a telephone in all fifty states and the District of Columbia. Only female interviewers surveyed women respondents. For men, approximately half of the interviews were conducted by women interviewers and half were conducted by male interviewers. A Spanish-language translation was administered by bilingual interviewers for Spanish-speaking respondents. The survey was introduced to respondents as a survey on "personal safety."

Sample

Of the 8,000 women surveyed, 6,312 women (78.9 percent of eligible respondents) were included in the analysis (other women were excluded because of essential missing information, such as sexual orientation and responses to key violence variables). Only women are examined in this analysis because the sample of men who detailed their experiences of violence and health care-seeking behaviors was too small to yield reliable results for the advanced statistical tests. However, this issue is addressed in the discussion section, as there is need for better research on men's experiences of violence.

Ages of women respondents ranged from eighteen to ninety-seven, with a mean age of forty-two years. Approximately 99 percent (6,233) of the respondents reported being heterosexual; of the remaining seventy-nine women (1.25 percent) who reported either being in a current same-sex relationship or having had a past same-sex relationship, eighteen had been in a relationship with both a man and a woman. Most (82 percent) respondents are white, followed by black (8 percent), mixed race (5 percent), Asian or Pacific Islander (2 percent), and lastly American Indian or Alaskan Native and "don't know" racial category (both just over 1 percent). Around 8 percent of respondents also reported being Hispanic. Income was fairly normally distributed, with most women reporting a yearly income between $5,000–50,000 (87 percent), but no women reporting making over $100,000 a year. Most respondents received at least a high school degree (89 percent), with 30 percent completing a four-year college degree and 26 percent completing postgraduate education. In terms of employment, just under half reported being employed full-time (48 percent), though 13.5 percent of women were only employed part-time and 17 percent self-identified as a homemaker. A detailed breakdown of demographic characteristics can be found in appendix A.

Data and Methods

To be succinct, IPV can be described as an *unwanted systemic set of ongoing behaviors that falls outside normative boundaries and spirals multidirectionally over time around issues of control and power with the intention of enhancing the perpetrator's power at the expense of the victim* (Lehman, 1997). With this idea of control and power in mind, three specific forms of abuse are most prominent within the domestic and intimate violence literature: physical, sexual, and emotional/psychological (which includes verbal abuse). Other abuse forms (intellectual, spiritual, intimate stalking, control, and use of the children) are largely ignored. Some argue that imposed social isolation and/or control is best considered itself as an independent form of violence given the frequency and impact with which it strikes (Stark, 2009).

This analysis examines physical, sexual, emotional (which includes verbal abuse), and control violence within two different types of relationships[5]: live-in spouses and partners, and live-apart boyfriend/girlfriend or dating partners (descriptive statistical information for these variables can be found in tables 9.1 and 9.2 in the results section).

This analysis seeks to better understand the health-related effects of IPV on individuals and their health-care-seeking behaviors. To measure health-related outcomes, variables were constructed that took into account the specific injuries received from the reported physical or sexual violence, as well as a person reporting psychological injury or emotional stress following physical or sexual violence. In addition, to measure the health-related effect of emotional violence, a life-stressors and depression scale was created using most of the variables within the survey's PTSD inventory[6] (descriptive statistics for these variables can be found in tables 9.3 and 9.4 in the results section).

Lastly, to measure health care behaviors, variables were constructed to indicate if a person sought out medical care, emergency services, or surgery for their physical injuries or psychological counseling/treatment (via licenses practitioner or conversations with a crisis hotline, victim's advocate, or support group) for their psychological injury or emotional stress (descriptive statistics for these variables can be found in tables 9.5 and 9.6 in the results section). Due to limitations with the survey, this analysis can examine only health care-seeking behaviors that directly follow physical and sexual violence.

Stata/SE 13 quantitative data analysis software for large datasets was used. The main statistical techniques in the analysis are descriptive and inferential (namely Fisher's Exact test for small frequencies), used to determine similarities and differences between groups (opposite-sex relationships and same-sex violence) in terms of violent experiences, health-related outcomes, and health care-seeking behaviors (Stevens, 2002).

RESULTS

Proposition #1: IPV is more prevalent in same-sex partnerships than opposite-sex partnerships.

The rates of IPV experienced by all women, regardless of relationship type, are high (though well within the expected ranges). Specifically, in Tables 9.1 and 9.2 below, we see that more than half of all women experience physical abuse, either by the men they live with (62.6 percent) or are dating (52 percent), or by the women they live with (68 percent) or are dating (50 percent). Slightly less women experience sexual violence, though the rates are still between one-quarter and one-half of all women: 22.5 percent of women experience sexual violence by a husband or live-in opposite-sex partner, while 48 percent experience sexual violence by a boyfriend or opposite-sex dating partner. Likewise, 31 percent of women experience sexual violence by a wife or live-in same-sex partner and 36.4 percent experience sexual violence by a girlfriend or dating partner.

We can also see that women in opposite-sex relationships experience emotional and control violence less often than women in same-sex relationships. Indeed, in opposite-sex relationships we see almost half of all women experiencing emotional violence (49.8 percent), and 37.4 percent detailing

Table 9.1. Descriptive Statistics for Intimate Violence in Opposite-Sex Relationships

		Percent Experienced	Mode	Minimum	Maximum	N
Physical Violence	Live-in Partner/Spouse	62.6%	1	0	1	1939
	Live-apart Boyfriend/Dating	51.9%	1	0	1	476
Sexual Violence	Live-in Partner/Spouse	22.5%	0	0	1	1175
	Live-apart Boyfriend/Dating	48.0%	0	0	1	560
Emotional Violence	Live-in Partner/Spouse	49.8%	0	0	1	5929
Control Violence	Live-in Partner/Spouse	37.4%	0	0	1	5929

Notes:
1) Emotional and control violence are measured only for live-in spouses or partners (past and current).
2) Mode 0=no violence, mode 1=violence
3) Sample size varies depending on how many women answered the questions. For all variables, nonresponses were coded as missing (".")
Source: U.S. Department of Justice, National Violence Against Women Survey, 1994–1996.

Table 9.2. Descriptive Statistics for Intimate Violence in Same-Sex Relationships

		Percent Experienced	Mode	Minimum	Maximum	N
Physical Violence	Live-in Partner/Spouse	68.3%	1	0	1	41
	Live-apart Girlfriend/Dating	50.0%	1	0	1	10
Sexual Violence	Live-in Partner/Spouse	31.0%	0	0	1	29
	Live-apart Girlfriend/Dating	36.4%	0	0	1	11
Emotional Violence	Live-in Partner/Spouse	74.7%	1	0	1	79
Control Violence	Live-in Partner/Spouse	67.1%	1	0	1	79

Notes:
1) Emotional and control violence are measured only for live-in spouses or partners (past and current).
2) Mode 0=no violence, mode 1=violence
3) Sample size varies depending on how many women answered the questions. For all variables, nonresponses were coded as missing (" .").
Source: U.S. Department of Justice, National Violence Against Women Survey, 1994–1996.

instances of control. However, women in same-sex relationships report much higher rates, with 75 percent experiencing emotional violence and 67 percent experiencing control.

The Fisher's Exact test (table 9.7 below) for differences between opposite-sex IPV and same-sex IPV shows us a more detailed side to this story. Although all women experience high rates of violence in their intimate partnerships, women in same-sex relationships experience emotional ($p<.001$) and control ($p<.001$) violence significantly more.

Proposition #2: The negative health outcomes of IPV affect all people, regardless of the sex/gender of the survivor or abuser.

In line with previous literature and the myriad physical and mental health outcomes of IPV, this analysis finds that more than one-quarter of women report having physical injuries from physical and/or sexual violence. Physical injuries that were reported included, but were not limited to, pregnancy-related outcomes (unwanted pregnancy, abortion, miscarriage), sexually transmitted diseases, spinal cord injuries, bullet wounds, burns, internal injuries, and psychological injury or emotional distress.

Tables 9.3 and 9.4 detail that on average, women in same-sex relationships reported negative health outcomes more often than women in opposite-sex relationships. For instance, 39.5 percent of women abused by their opposite-sex partners reported physical injuries after the most recent physical violence experience, while 48.7 percent of women abused by same-sex partners did. Additionally, 27.5 percent of women abused by an opposite-sex partner reported physical injuries after the most recent sexual violence experience, while 35.7 percent of women abused by a same-sex partner did.

Psychological injury and emotional stress were no different. Under 2 percent of both women in opposite-sex relationships and same-sex relationships reported emotional distress after the most recent physical violence they experienced, while 4.4 percent of women abused by men and 16.7 percent of women abused by women reported emotional distress following the most recent sexual violence experience. The PTSD inventory, which measured a person's week-previous emotional and/or depressive state of mind, finds that 100 percent of all women reported at least some level of distress or depression because of the violence they have experienced by a spouse, partner, or dating partner, with the mean response being slightly higher for women abused by women (indicating slightly more distress/depression).

The Fisher's Exact test (table 9.7 below) for differences shows us, however, that women in opposite-sex and same-sex relationships are experiencing negative health outcomes at similar rates. Indeed, none of the physical or emotional health variables differed significantly based on the sex/gender of the abusive partner.

Table 9.3. Health- and Mental Health-Related Effects of Intimate Partner Violence in Opposite-Sex Relationships

		Percent Experienced	Mode/Mean	Minimum	Maximum	N
Physical Violence	Physical Injuries	39.5%	0	0	1	1705
	Psychological Stress	1.8%	0	0	1	674
Sexual Violence	Physical Injuries	27.5%	0	0	1	1138
	Psychological Stress	4.4%	0	0	1	293
Emotional & Control Violence	Life Stress/Depression Inventory	100.0%	10.2	5	79	6233

Notes:
1) Mode is used for binary 0/1 variables; mean is used for interval/scale variables.
2) Mode 0=no injury(ies), mode 1=injury(ies)
3) The PTSD Inventory used in the survey has a possible range of 1 (for no stress/depression reported) to 5 (for maximum amount of stress/depression reported), for each of twenty total questions.
4) All women in the survey reported some level of stress related to violence in her current relationship.
5) Sample size varies depending on how many women answered the questions. For all variables, nonresponses were coded as missing (".").
Source: U.S. Department of Justice, National Violence Against Women Survey, 1994–1996.

Table 9.4. Health- and Mental Health-Related Effects of Intimate Partner Violence in Same-Sex Relationships

		Percent Experienced	Mode/Mean	Minimum	Maximum	N
Physical Violence	Physical Injuries	48.7%	0	0	1	37
	Psychological Stress	0.0%	0	0	0	18
Sexual Violence	Physical Injuries	35.7%	0	0	1	28
	Psychological Stress	16.7%	0	0	1	12
Emotional & Control Violence	Life Stress/Depression Inventory	100.0%	10.8	9	60	79

Notes:
1) Mode is used for binary 0/1 variables; mean is used for interval/scale variables.
2) Mode 0=no injury(ies), mode 1=injury(ies)
3) The PTSD Inventory used in the survey has a possible range of 1 (for no stress/depression reported) to 5 (for maximum amount of stress/depression reported), for each of twenty total questions.
4) All women in the survey reported some level of stress related to violence in her current relationship.
5) Sample size varies depending on how many women answered the questions. For all variables, nonresponses were coded as missing (" ").
Source: U.S. Department of Justice, National Violence Against Women Survey, 1994–1996.

Proposition #3: Those who experience same-sex IPV seek out and use physical and mental health care services less often than those who experience opposite-sex IPV.

Although high rates of physical and sexual violence occur for all women in the sample, on average, only 30 percent or fewer women seek out physical and/or psychological health care services. In this survey, physical medical care includes hospital and emergency room visits, special surgeries for injuries suffered, outpatient services (i.e., physical therapy), and/or home care, among other assistances. Psychological health care services included reporting discussing the event with a licensed psychiatrist, psychologist, social worker, crisis hotline and/or victim's advocate, support group, or "mental health professional."

Tables 9.5 and 9.6 show that after the most recent experience of physical violence, 32 percent of women abused by men and 11 percent of women abused by women sought out medical care services, while 23.2 percent of women abused by men and 29.7 percent of women abused by women sought out psychological care services.

For the most recent sexual violence experience, 14.2 percent of women abused by men and 11.5 percent of women abused by women received medical care, while 6.1 percent of women abused by men and 20.3 percent of women abused by women were treated by or discussed the violence with a psychological service care provider.

The Fisher's Exact test (table 9.7 below) reveals some particularly interesting results. For physical violence, women abused by men are significantly more likely than women abused by women to seek out medical care ($p=.044$) but equally likely to seek out psychological care. However, for sexual violence, although all woman are equally likely to seek out (or in this case, *not* seek out) medical care, women abused by women are significantly more likely than women abused by men to seek out psychological care ($p<.001$). Thus, even though around one-third of women in opposite-sex relationships seek out both psychological and medical care services following physical violence, significantly fewer women (11 percent) in same-sex relationships seek out medical care following a physically violent event. Contrarily, fewer than 20 percent of women seek out psychological or medical care services following sexual violence, but women in same-sex relationships seek out psychological care significantly more often.

It should also be noted that just over 200 women in opposite-sex relationships and five women in same-sex relationships reported having told their medical care provider about the exact nature of the injuries they received after their physical or sexual violence experience (see tables 9.5 and 9.6). So even though, on average, almost half of women experienced physical or sexual violence by an

Table 9.5. Health-Care-Seeking Behaviors of Survivors after Violence in Opposite-Sex Relationships

		Percent Experienced	Mode	Minimum	Maximum	N
Physical Violence	Medical care	32.1%	0	0	1	674
	Psychological care	23.2%	0	0	1	1705
	Discussed nature of physical injuries with medical care provider?	20.3%	1	0	1	212
Sexual Violence	Medical care	14.2%	0	0	1	841
	Psychological care	6.1%	0	0	1	6233
	Discussed nature of physical injuries with medical care provider?	8.9%	1	0	1	106

Notes:
1) Mode 0=did not seek care; mode 1=did seek care
2) Sample size varies depending on how many women answered the questions. For all variables, nonresponses were coded as missing (".").
Source: U.S. Department of Justice, National Violence Against Women Survey, 1994–1996.

Table 9.6. Health-Care-Seeking Behaviors of Survivors after Violence in Same-Sex Relationships

		Percent Experienced	Mode	Minimum	Maximum	N
Physical Violence	Medical care	11.1%	0	0	1	18
	Psychological care	29.7%	0	0	1	37
	Discussed nature of physical injuries with medical care provider?	11.1%	1	0	1	3
Sexual Violence	Medical care	11.5%	0	0	1	26
	Psychological care	20.3%	0	0	1	79
	Discussed nature of physical injuries with medical care provider?	11.5%	1	0	1	2

Notes:
1) Mode 0=did not seek care; mode 1=did seek care
2) Sample size varies depending on how many women answered the questions. For all variables, nonresponses were coded as missing ("."),
Source: U.S. Department of Justice, National Violence Against Women Survey, 1994–1996.

Table 9.7. Fisher's Exact Tests for Differences in Outcomes between Women in Opposite-Sex and Same-Sex Relationships

		Fisher's p	N
Physical Violence	Live-in Partner/Spouse	0.281	1980
	Live-apart Boyfriend/Dating	0.587	486
	Physical Injuries	0.17	1742
	Psychological Stress	0.727	692
	Medical care	.044*	692
	Psychological care	0.228	1742
	Live-in Partner/Spouse	0.191	1204
	Live-apart Boyfriend/Dating	0.324	571
	Physical Injuries	0.221	1661
Sexual Violence	Psychological Stress	0.112	305
	Medical care	0.491	867
	Psychological care	>.001***	6312
Emotional Violence	Live-in Partner/Spouse	>.001***	6008
Control Violence	Live-in Partner/Spouse	>.001***	6008
Emotional and Control Violence	Life Stress/Depression Inventory	-.557	6312

Notes:

* $p < .05$

** $p < .01$

*** $p < .001$

1) Fisher's Exact test calculates the exact probability of the table being as unevenly distributed as observed given independence of rows and columns.

2) The number for "Live Stress/Depression Inventory" is a z-test statistic for the Mann-Whitney test, used for independent samples with ordinal-level data.

Source: U.S. Department of Justice, National Violence Against Women Survey, 1994–1996.

intimate partner, only an average of 22 percent of women abused by men and 11 percent of women abused by women told their care service provider exactly how they had received their physical injuries.

DISCUSSION

This analysis set out to add to the slowly growing body of literature on IPV as a health issue. Even more, this analysis was aimed at identifying the differing experiences of women abused by men and women abused by women. Previous nationally representative research had, to this point, revealed that a higher percentage of women who identify as lesbian and/or bisexual (or who report same-sex sexual and intimate relationships) experience violence by a current or former intimate partner than heterosexually identified women (or women who report opposite-sex sexual and intimate relationships). However, these analyses and reports stopped short of testing for statistically significant differences between these groups utilizing a representative, probability sample. We were left to wonder how much more violence a lesbian or bisexual woman has to experience in order to be experiencing it significantly more often and whether or not the outcomes were disparate.

This study confirms that for some types of violence and some healthcare-seeking behaviors, sexual orientation does matter, though, perhaps not as we might expect. For this sample, women abused by women were significantly more likely to experience emotional and control violence and significantly more likely to seek out psychological care after a sexual violence experience. However, women abused by women were also significantly less likely to seek out medical care for physical injuries after a physical violence experience.

While some might jump to making a gender-normative argument about why women are perpetrating emotional and control violence against their partners more often than men (i.e., women are more emotional in general, jealous, possessive, yell instead of fight physically, etc.), there may be another plausible explanation: minority stress. Minority stress is a concept based on the premise that LGBT people in a heterosexist society are subjected to chronic stress related to their stigmatization (Meyer, 1995). This stress can be directly related to the rejection, discrimination, and violence they experience in everyday life, but it can also manifest because of internalized homophobia (projecting society's negative views of you inwards toward yourself). Studies have shown that minority stress has numerous mental health effects, such as depression and distress, but also feelings of helplessness and anger (Meyer, 1995). In the end, the result of this distress and anger is often lower relationship quality, higher levels of arguing and fighting, and in some cases, the desire to keep secret your own sexual orientation or relationship, and/or control your significant other's contact with the outside world (Balsam, 2001; Balsam & Szymanski, 2005; Mohr & Daly, 2008; Otis, Rostosky, Riggle, & Hamrin, 2006). More research is needed to confirm this proposition, namely a comparative study with men to see if the same trends in emotional and control violence are discerned, and additional qualitative data, which has the power to ask more targeted questions related to minority stress, mental health, relationship quality, and violence types.

We must also take note that although women abused by women were not physically or sexually victimized significantly more often than women abused by men, all women experienced equally high rates of this violence, with 50 to 68 percent reporting physical violence and 22 to 48 percent reporting sexual violence. It's not, to put it simply, as if women are only abusing their intimate partners emotionally and with use of control tactics.

Although the second finding on health care utilization is consistent with the barriers to access and lacking cultural competency framework, the first (women abused by women seeking psychological care following sexual violence more often) is not. What might explain lesbian and bisexual women's seeking out psychological care lies in the demographic characteristics of the sample. In this sample, lesbian and bisexual women are significantly older, have a higher level of education, are more likely to be employed full-time, and make more money. Given that psychological care is often expensive and/or requires decent medical/insurance coverage, it is not surprising that those most likely to seek psychological care would be those who are employed full time or making more money. Beyond that, there is a social stigma attached to seeking out psychological care that has been shown to be less strong for older and more educated individuals, who tend to seek out psychological care more often than younger, less-educated individuals (Gonzalez, Alegria, Prihoda, Copeland, & Zeber, 2011; Surgenor, 1985).

This analysis also highlights the ineffectuality of the health care system in scanning for and treating IPV, as well as women's general experience of nonreporting. For instance, only 11 percent of women abused by women sought out medical care for their injuries in the first place (although the women who sought out this care did discuss the nature of their injuries with those providers). Of the 674 women abused physically by men, only 31 percent discussed the nature of their injuries with the medical care provider who treated them; even fewer (12.6 percent) discussed their experience of intimate sexual violence. If a woman responded that she did not discuss the nature of her injuries with the medical care provider, it could be because the provider did not ask her how it happened or it could be that the provider asked, but the woman did not want to discuss the violence against her. This analysis thus confirms that health care service providers aren't asking the right questions and/or women are lying about the causes and circumstances of their injuries.

There are, however, limitations to this current study. The main one has to do with the age of the survey. The reasoning behind the choice to use the National Violence Against Women Survey (NVAWS) data is mostly practical: There are no other representative surveys available for use that fulfill all the qualifications for this analysis (myriad types of violence, sexual orientation variable, identification of perpetrator's sex/gender and the nature of their relationship to you, questions about health). All of the data is ruled out (The National Crime Victimization Survey, The Conflict and Tactics Scale when used with no demographic supplement, the National Intimate Partner and Sexual Violence Survey, Behavioral Risk Factor Surveillance System data, the General Social Survey, National Survey of Family and Households, California Health Interview Survey), except for the NVAWS.

Another limitation is the small sample of women who identify as having current or former relationships with women. Some have argued that a behaviorally based way of identifying sexual orientation is ineffective, and a self-identified categorical response should be used instead. However, although researchers and demographers know that the self-reported LGB population is somewhere in the range of 3 to 5 percent of the entire population (Gates, 2011), surveys that categorize individuals based on behaviors, such as cohabitation, see much lower response rates. According to the U.S. Census Bureau, in 2008 there were 230,117,876 Americans aged eighteen or older and 564,743, or 0.25 percent, were cohabitating with a partner of the same-sex (O'Connell & Lofquist, 2009). Of the original NVAWS sample of 16,000 Americans aged eighteen or older, 58 or 0.36 percent of respondents were cohabitating with a same-sex partner at the time of the survey. Based solely on same-sex cohabitation rates, the NVAWS closely mirrors the population.

In general, there is a great need for better data on same-sex violence and LGBT health. Future research should take into account: increased sampling of men (barriers can be particularly bad for gay and transgender men) (Jeffries & Ball, 2008; Kay & Jeffries, 2010; Merrill & Wolfe, 2000); increased sampling of diverse populations (the women in the survey, for example, were mostly white, non-Hispanic, moderately educated, middle class, working, and reasonably healthy); and more focused studies of emotional and control violence, which effect a large proportion of women and of which we do not fully understand the physical and psychological effects.

CONCLUSION

Today, because of the hard work of researchers and academics, the National Institute of Health now includes LGBT individuals as a specific minority health population (they join the other traditionally included subpopulations: youth and young adults, minority populations, people of low income, people with low educational attainment, and people with mental health or medical comorbidities).

However, unlike the adverse effects of smoking or alcoholism (a popular focus for LGBT health researchers) or other commonly cited general health issues like obesity, cancer, or depression, IPV remains a seemingly controversial issue. More than *individual* vices or diseases, IPV threatens the social and moral fabric of relationships and families. Those against LGBT equality can point to same-sex violence as a reason for upholding inequity, and those for equality can desire same-sex violence to be kept silent as to avoid any negative associations with LGBT relationships and families. This veil of silence keeps the issue of same-sex IPV in the closet, leaving the very people who need care the most severely unprotected.

Same-sex and LGBT IPV is a critical health issue that can no longer be ignored. According to the Human Rights Campaign, speaking on the drafting of the latest edit to the Violence Against Women Act (which originally failed to pass because of its inclusion of LGBT protections):

> "During the process of soliciting information to draft the Senate bill, it became clear that LGBT victims of domestic violence were not receiving the services they needed—even though they experience domestic violence at roughly the same rate as all other victims. LGBT victims faced discrimination based on their sexual orientation and gender identity when they sought refuge from abuse. They were turned away from service providers, laughed at by law enforcement, and struggled to get protective orders from judges. Often they were left without any option but to return to their abuser."

NOTES

1. Violence Against Women Act. http://frwebgate.access.gpo.gov/cgi-bin/getdoc.cgi?dbname=109_cong_bills&docid=f:h3402enr.txt.pdf.

2. For example, individuals are often recruited at local community centers, at LGBT events, such as Pride marches, and via email listserves and snowball sampling (Balsam et al., 2005; Balsam & Szymanski, 2005).

3. "Heterosexism" describes "an ideological system that denies, denigrates, and stigmatizes any nonheterosexual form of behavior, identity, relationship or community."

Gregory M. Herek, "The Context of anti-gay violence: Notes on cultural and psychological heterosexism, *"Journal of Interpersonal Violence*, No. 5, pp. 316–333. http://psychology.ucdavis.edu/rainbow/html/prej_defn.html#Herek90_txt.

4. Here, the term describes an environment in which individuals' "gender identity [is expected to] correspond to their birth-assigned sex and/or stereotypes associated with that sex." 2005. Transgender Law Center, "10 Tips for Working with Transgender Individuals. A guide for health care providers." www.transgenderlawcenter.org.

5. More specific information on variable construction is available upon request.

6. It should be noted that these questions were about any and all violence, including physical and sexual, experienced by a person's current spouse/partner and is measured as stressful and depressive thoughts experienced within the last seven days.

Political Activism as a
Heath-Giving Activity

Transforming Silence into Language and Action

Michael Warren Tumolo

$\mathcal{A}$udre Lorde began her talk at the meeting of the Modern Language Association in 1977 by explaining how confronting breast cancer made her realize much of what she understands about the "transformation of silence into language and action" (Lorde, 1984, p. 40). Those who differ from societal norms, Lorde explains, live in "silence," fearful of "contempt, of censure, or some judgment, or recognition, of challenge, of annihilation" (p. 42). Such fears of being "audible" may systematically disempower individuals, leaving them passive victims who have voices, yet never give voice. This inner experience of silence is met by external experiences in which multiple forms of discriminatory silencing are used against individuals or groups marked as different from some cultural norms, however arbitrary those norms may be.

From the rhetorical perspective that this essay assumes, avowing that an individual or group has been silenced indicates that they have been stripped of rhetorical agency or otherwise disempowered. This essay goes further by arguing that silence targeting LGBT communities makes people ill: Silence kills. Although silence does have negative consequences on people's health and well-being, it can also be a resource for positive change. As Michel Foucault (1990) notes, silence is "an element that functions alongside the things said, with them and in relation to them within overall strategies"; it stands as a resource for resistance to the health consequences engendered by acts of silencing (p. 27). It is in this context that we may broaden our understanding of political activism by considering some forms of political activism as health-giving activities. This essay addresses how silence is used both to discriminate against and to empower LGBT people in the context of scholarly literature on the health consequences of anti-LGBT discrimination.

METHODS

This essay's critical and theoretical approach is guided by Brett Lunceford's (2011) call for rhetorical scholarship to reach back to the early roots of the discipline and address contemporary issues that are relevant and timely for scholarly and lay audiences. Michael Tumolo (2011) similarly argues that this perspective on rhetorical scholarship calls for rhetorical scholarship to be "brought to bear on immediate social, cultural, and political contexts" (p. 55). Lunceford notes that rhetorical scholarship often addresses historical issues because it is "only with hindsight that the rhetorician can proclaim the importance of the discourse" and make claims about the discourse's presumed effects (p. 3). Historical rhetorical scholarship, Lunceford explains, is able to operate closer to a social scientific paradigm in which the historical archive stands surrogate for empirical data. Such an archive is not available for contemporary issues in which the chain of events is ongoing. In such cases, rhetorical scholarship takes on the function of identifying discourses in need of address, demonstrating their inner-animating logics, and calling for additional scrutiny. Barry Brummett (1984) has thus offered an explanation of rhetorical scholarship as being designed "to teach people how to experience their rhetorical environments more richly" (p. 103). The rhetorical environment includes immediately recognizable forms of rhetorical address (i.e., speeches, music, films, and websites) and contextual determinates (i.e., previous knowledge, attitudes, and values). In the interplay between texts and contexts, rhetorical scholars Robert J. Branham and W. Barnett Pearce (1985) explain that "every communicative act is a text that derives meaning from the context of expectations and constraints in which it is experienced" (p. 19). In focusing on contemporary discourses that have not yet met some form of historical terminus, rhetorical scholarship draws attention to contemporary discourses while revealing how and with what consequences that these discourses operate in our rhetorical culture.

This essay demonstrates how silence is used in contradictory ways to both discriminate against and support the health and well-being of LGBT individuals and communities. As an instance of contemporary rhetorical scholarship, this essay demonstrates how a set of discourses and practices serve to repress and/or empower LGBT people. To this end, this essay works at two levels of abstraction, one highly local and one global, to establish a clear image of the ultimate health consequence of anti-LGBT discrimination: the destruction of life. This part of the essay draws attention to the underreported[1] killing of Sakia Gunn, whose killer was found guilty of committing a crime with the "purpose to intimidate an individual or group because of sexual orientation," which is a testament to how systemic discrimination has demonstrable consequences on the health and well-being of LGBT people (Meenan, 2003a, para. 1). To put this incident into context, the Southern Poverty Law Center offers an online resource for accessing details of the "approximately 191,000 reported and unreported hate crimes" occurring each year in the United States (2013, para. 1). The most recent statistics compiled by the Federal Bureau of Investigation (2011) indicate that 20.5 percent of those hate crimes reported to the FBI were motivated by antihomosexual bias.

Recognizing that epistemic demands of scholarship require more than empathic responses to an individual case, this local discourse is framed in terms of broad scholarly research on psychological and physiological health conse- quences of a culture of anti-LGBT discrimination. At this level of abstraction, the essay demonstrates how a set of extraordinary health consequences results from crimes of commission (intentional acts) as well as omission (failure to act). On the global level, this essay addresses an international activist move- ment that turns silence on its head by challenging silence's effects on LGBT people and serving as a source of empowerment. The essay explains key stra- tegic discourses developed as part of the National Day of Silence Project to demonstrate how it works as a corrective that contributes to the health and well-being of LGBT people.

RESULTS

Beyond issues of political and rhetorical representation, the consequences of systemic silencing strike at the core of LGBT people's health and well-being. This essay demonstrates ways that "silence" has been used as a tool *by*, *for*, and *against* lesbian, gay, bisexual, and transgender individuals and communities. Whereas bias intimidation killings represent the extreme consequences of sys- temic anti-LGBT discrimination, standing research on the topic demonstrates how the negative health consequences are far more varied and pervasive. Further, it shows how activists' calls for justice may impact the health of the community. The most chilling aspect of the research shows how the most prevalent crimes are ones of omission rather than commission, characterized by the failure to action in the realms of government, education, and the law. Such omission has produced a phenomenon that critics have labeled "death by denial" in response to government research that found LGBT youths to be four times more likely to commit suicide than their straight peers (Feinleib, 1989). This increased likelihood is significant given that the Center for Disease Control (2010) reports suicide as the number-two cause of death for youths ages ten to twenty-four in its most recent data concerning the leading causes of death (unintentional injury is the leading cause for this age-group).

In summary, findings include:

- Silence is a rhetorical strategy used to both disempower and empower LGBT individuals and communities.
- Silencing brings with it a host of psychological and physiological effects, ranging from psychosocial maladjustment to suicide and murder.
- In the specific case of LGBT youth suicide, the most significant contributing factors are communicative acts including bullying, name-calling, and harassment.
- Cultural norms of discrimination against LGBT individuals and communities foster violence against LGBT individuals and acts of self-harm.
- Pro-LGBT activism may mitigate the consequences of anti-LGBT silencing.

These findings are drawn from the literature and case studies addressed in the following discussion section.

DISCUSSION

Two cases in which silence is transformed into language and action elucidate how political activism may serve as a health-giving activity. The first case personalizes the issue by addressing the victim of one hate crime in the context of a growing body of literature on the health consequences of anti-LGBT victimization. The second case examines how a longstanding international protest movement has developed and refined its challenge to anti-LGBT discrimination.

Health Consequences of Anti-LGBT Victimization: Murder, Suicide, and Psychological Ailments

On Tuesday, May 13, 2003: *The New York Times* reported that a "15–year–old girl returning with four friends from a party in Manhattan was fatally stabbed at a bus stop [in Newark, New Jersey] early Sunday morning during a scuffle with two men whose advances the girls rebuffed" (Smothers, 2003a, p. 8). One day later, the Newark police issued a warrant for twenty-nine–year-old Richard McCullough, who they believed was involved in this fatal stabbing (Kelley, 2003, p. 5). On that Friday, McCullough went with his lawyer to the Essex County prosecutors' office to turn himself in (Smothers, 2003b, p. 4). He was arraigned on murder, weapons possession, and a bias intimidation charge. He entered a not-guilty plea to all the charges.

Three days earlier, on Saturday, May 10, 2003, Sakia Gunn and her friends headed from their homes in Newark, New Jersey, to the Christopher Street pier in Manhattan's West Village. Her friend Victoria Dingle explained that "the pier is somewhere we go to feel open about ourselves and have fun. . . . Me and Sakia and some friends were just chilling and having fun and feeling good about being together" (Cianciotto & Cahill, 2003, p. 86). Victoria took a cab home; the rest took the train to Newark and waited for a bus around three in the morning. One of the witnesses remembered two men driving up in a white car, one shouting, "Yo, Shorty. Come here" (Cianciotto & Cahill, p. 87).

The men wanted something that the lesbian youths did not intend to give. The words they exchanged did not please the men: "One girl told them they were not interested because they were lesbians" (Kelley, 2003, p. 5). During the altercation that followed, McCullough allegedly got out of the car and grabbed Kahmya Woodbridge by the neck. She was released when Sakia fought back. Sakia was stabbed in the chest and died at the emergency room that night. After a six-month-long investigation, the Essex County prosecutors' indicted McCullough on six charges, including "murder with a purpose to intimidate an individual or group because of sexual orientation" (Meenan, 2003a, para. 1). The charges were reduced from second-degree murder as part of a plea agreement, and he pleaded guilty to aggravated manslaughter, aggravated assault, and bias intimidation and was sentenced to twenty years in prison (Meenan, 2005).

This story is about more than an isolated act of murder. The actions of the principal of West Side High School where Sakia was enrolled in the tenth grade indicate the pervasiveness of the kind of mentality that led to Gunn's death. Several students in the school alleged that Principal Williams "refused to declare a moment of silence for Sakia" saying that "if someone chooses to live a certain lifestyle, they must pay a certain price" (Cianciotto & Cahill, 2003, p. 87–88; Fouratt, 2003). This educator's response sent a chilling message by erroneously claiming that sexual orientation is a matter of choice and that such a choice warrants death. In this logic, Gunn's sexual orientation was enough to revoke the minor solace provided by brief public mourning. Rather than normalizing compassion, the response revealed existing norms of discrimination against LGBT people.

Sadly, this discrimination is not isolated. To greater or lesser degrees, this is consistent with the discriminatory messages that educators and educational staff are targeting LGBT youths with across the country. In a nationwide poll, 56.9 percent of LGBT youths had heard educators or educational staff make homophobic remarks and negative remarks about gender expression (Kosciw, Greytak, Bartiewicz, Boesen, & Palmer, 2012, p. xiv). Further, of youths who reported being physically harassed, verbally harassed, or physically assaulted, only 39.6 percent reported the incidents and of those reports, 36.7 percent indicated that the staff did nothing in response (Kosciw et al., p. xv). The actions of the killer and the educator are in line with numerous cultural practices that lead to the same result: the untimely death of LGBT youths.

In 1989, the U.S. Department of Health and Human Services found that lesbian, gay, and bisexual youths are four times more likely to commit suicide than their straight peers (Feinleib, 1989). Anti-LGBT advocates have used these studies to argue that LGBT individuals are fundamentally flawed; however, instead of supporting these biases, these studies provide support for something far more sinister, namely that there are many mitigating factors that stand behind such a high correlation between sexual orientation and suicide. The studies show a significantly higher rate of suicide for heterosexuals and homosexuals who remain abstinent. They also show psychosocial factors such as intolerance, name-calling, harassment, and exclusion (not sexual orientation) to be the main determinates of suicidal ideation (thinking or planning), suicide attempts, and suicide. With the lines drawn as such, these findings suggest that antidiscrimination policies and sexual wellness education would directly contribute to the health of the nation's youth. Instead of action, however, the administration chose silence, consequently promoting a culture of "death by denial" leading to the unnecessary suicides of many homosexual youths (Remafedi, 1994). These findings are broadly supported by research on risk factors facing LGBT youths, with the consensus identifying environmental factors including victimization, harassment, and bullying as primary causes for suicide, suicide ideation, and suicide attempts (D'Augelli, Grossman, Salter, Vasey, Starks, & Sinclair, 2005; Johnson, Oxendine, Taub, & Robertson, 2013; Halady, 2013; Mustanski & Liu, 2013).

Suicide is a particularly powerful indicator of the severity of the problem insofar as it signifies the end point of a volatile chain reaction that features numerous health consequences that pale in comparison. Johnson et al. (2013) draw on previous research to demonstrate how vulnerability, victimization, mental health, and suicide intersect (p. 61). In their explanation, lesbian, gay, and bisexual people are vulnerable due to cultural attitudes toward their sexual orientation, and transgender people are vulnerable due to their gender expression. In the type of culture where even the majority of educators openly discriminate against LGBT people, this vulnerability invites victimization, which results in new or exacerbated instances of "depression, decreased self-esteem, decreased self-worth, feelings of entrapment, loneliness, withdrawal, anxiety, insomnia, hopelessness . . ." (Johnson et al., p. 61). Victimization encompasses a range of behaviors including verbal, psychological, and physical abuse, and may happen in the context of bullying (Swearer, Turner, Givens, & Pollack, 2008; Sourander et al., 2007, Bond, Carlin, Thomas, Rubin, & Patton, 2001). The range of health consequences include post-traumatic stress disorder (PTSD) (D'Augelli, Grossman, & Starks, 2006; Rivers 2004), psychosocial maladjustment (Eisenberg & Aalsma, 2005; Hawker & Boulton, 2000; Russell, Ryan, Toomey, Diaz, & Sanchez, 2011; Toomey, Ryan, Diaz, Card, & Russell, 2010), and increased health risk behaviors (Bontempo & D'Augelli, 2002; Bossarte, Swahn, & Breiding, 2009). In sum, a culture that allows for the largely unchecked victimization of LGBT youths produces a set of conditions that have potentially devastating health consequences on the community, ranging from psychological traumas to suicide and murder.

Thus far, this essay has demonstrated four forms of silence imposed on LGBT communities. They are as follows: the crime that condemned Sakia to the silence of the grave; the victimization represented by her high school principal and those educators and educational staff whose action and words demean the lived experiences of LGBT youths; a presidential administration's denial of the health and well-being of LGBT youths; and a range of psychosocial health consequences emerging from the overall context of anti-LGBT victimization. The message leaking through suggests that, rather than providing an environment built on discourses of political rights to nurture individual and collective excellence, American culture is aligned to promote sickness, decay, and death, particularly in vulnerable populations.

In the context of systemic victimization, LGBT communities have a difficult time legitimating their own narratives, which limits their ability to build rhetorical agency. This does not mean to suggest some sort of essential metanarrative governing LGBT experiences. As Johnson et al. (2013) succinctly put it, "being a member of the LGBT community or a victim of bullying does not automatically mean that one will become engaged in suicidal behavior" (p. 61). By contrast, the data suggests that a culture promoting anti-LGBT discourses and actions has demonstrable negative health consequences.

In this context where identifiable facets of a culture create a multitude of problems, political activism may be directed at changing the environmental risk factors while promoting protective factors to prevent health consequences. It is in this light that the tragedy of Sakia Gunn's murder reflected some promise for better tomorrows. One day prior to Gunn's funeral, two to three hundred people rallied outside of Newark's City Hall. They demanded that the mayor take an official stance in support of the identity represented by Sakia and against the hatred represented by her murder. The mayor did not meet with the people rallying, rendering their actions invisible through the depersonalization of his ignorance, aversion, or omission. This silencing fueled the sentiments driving the community that lost Sakia.

Friday, May 16, 2003: Reporter Jim Fouratt of the *Gay City News* arrived at the Perry Funeral Home in Newark, New Jersey. His eyes focused on a scene of around 2,500 people, mostly African American teenagers, surrounding a one-story building. He notices that the teens are "wearing rainbow colors everywhere they can bead, braid, paint, weave, stitch, and sew" (Fouratt, 2003, para. 2). He estimates that they are "90% lesbian between 14 and 16, and mourning the death of one of their gay girl sisters," who was "the butch cherub who had come to the defense of her friend when a couple of black men drove by and made a pass, one refusing to be rebuffed." They were waiting to pay tribute to Gunn, whose body lay still inside the building. The last words Fouratt recalled "were shouted at [him] from the organizer of the local HIV program that serves gay male teens, 'Don't forget about Sakia. Don't forget about us'" (para. 22). Lacquetta Nelson, former president of the New Jersey Stonewall Democrats, described the experience: "Never, in all my years of activism, have I ever witnessed anything as astounding as this" (Meenan, 2003b, para. 40).

The mourners at Sakia's funeral transformed her silence into visible action in a way that Mayor Sharpe James could not ignore. By provoking a protest, Sakia's final silence—death—gave voice to a community that is all too often silenced by hatred, oppression, and discrimination. The government officials were as unprepared for these teens taking to the streets as they were unaware of the magnitude of the impact made by Sakia's death on her community. Adolph St. Arromand, the project manager of Project WOW! Youth Center, a Newark-based HIV prevention group, helped assist and console many of the youths mourning at the funeral before the city sent in a crisis intervention unit (Meenan, 2003b). Mayor James was greeted coldly when he arrived at around 1:30 p.m. As he pledged that he would set up a "gay and lesbian counseling center in Gunn's name," masses of the teenagers walked out in protest (Meenan, 2003b, para. 47). They had not forgotten his inaction in front of City Hall and saw his pledge as being too little and too late for their deceased friend. Arromand noted that, "Maybe it took the death of Sakia for the world to see the truth" (Meenan 2003b, para. 26).

The people seized rhetorical agency when they transformed the silencing of Sakia into language and action. This story of activism was, however, largely contained. In the eleven months following the events, Gunn's murder was covered twenty-eight times compared to the 735 articles featuring Matthew Shepard over the same period of time (Pearson, 2006, p. 169). *The New York Times* carried the story of Sakia's murder without mentioning the civic engagement witnessed at her funeral. The later articles referred to the candlelight vigils and the demonstration in front of City Hall that the mayor responded to with silence, but the spectacle of Sakia's funeral was not mentioned. This omission may be brushed off as typical fare, yet the funeral was atypical given the 2,500 mourners that required the city to deploy a sizable crisis-intervention unit including ambulances, police, counselors, and food provisions (Smothers, 2003b, p. 4). In the mainstream press, Sakia's story was told with a cold efficiency. By contrast, in New York's *Gay City News*, Sakia's story was told with compassion and care with particular attention to the visual force of people coalescing at her funeral. Both presses make Sakia's story visible. The former provides an account whose sensation is not meant to last; the latter asks us to remember and to act.

Developing a Challenge to Anti-LGBT Discrimination: The National Day of Silence's Calculated Transformation of Silence into Language and Action

The tragic loss of Sakia Gunn offers a call to conscience that draws attention to the consequences of unchecked anti–LGBT discrimination. Standing scholarship indicates that this is not a localized issue involving isolated cases (i.e., Sakia Gunn and Matthew Shepard) that sometimes receive significant amounts of news coverage. Rather, the multiple silences imposed on LGBT people have predictable patterns of physical and psychological impact on youths and are entirely preventable. Programs and policies combatting these ill effects have proven effective in a variety of contexts (Espelage, Aragon, Birkett, & Koenig, 2008; Rienzo, Button, Sheu, & Li, 2006; Szalacha, 2003; Kosciw et al., 2011). The specific context of the bias intimidation murder draws attention to how the normalization of anti–LGBT discrimination fosters a range of behaviors and policies that promote victimization, resulting in issues with psychosocial adjustment, psychological trauma, suicide, and murder. The aftermath of this particular case focuses our attention on an even more important lesson— namely, that political activism may use such silences as the foundation upon which to provoke change for the health of the community.

The National Day of Silence Project is an exemplary international protest that addresses and challenges the damaging effects of silence on LGBT communities. The project's annual event, the National Day of Silence, is designed to provoke a transformation of silence into language as a resource for calling attention to and changing problems in American culture that lead to the host of health consequences previously addressed. The primary difference between this form of political activism and the protest at the memorial service discussed above is that the National Day of Silence is not an ad hoc event but rather a stable movement that has been refined over the years to make "silence" an effective mode of rhetorical tactic. This section offers a history of the project followed by a discussion of key organizational materials to show how it harnesses silence as a rhetorical resource for promoting cultural and political change that would promote the health and well-being of the LGBT community.

In 1996, eighteen-year-old Maria Pulzetti conceptualized the Day of Silence Project in an undergraduate essay at the University of Virginia. That year, 150 students at the University of Virginia held the first Day of Silence. Aided by extensive press coverage and a web page, the protest became a more significant phenomenon in 1997 with roughly one hundred schools participating (Gay, Lesbian, and Straight Education Network [GLSEN], 2011b, para. 1–4). Following this event, the project received endorsements from a number of significant humanitarian organizations, including the National Gay and Lesbian Task Force, the Human Rights Campaign, GLSEN, and the United Federation of Metropolitan Community Churches.

By 2001, the organizers had built a foundation of proven support, developed an institutional history, and displayed growth potential in high schools and colleges worldwide (GLSEN, 2011b, para. 1–6). GLSEN became an official organizational sponsor, bringing the project new funding, staff, and volunteers. At the same time, the organizers built a partnership with the United States Student Association (USSA) (GLSEN, 2011b, para. 7). Based in Washington, DC, the USSA is the oldest and largest national student association whose services include tracking and lobbying federal legislation and helping students collectively organize. The project additionally received broader public support from the likes of twenty-nine members of Congress who cosigned a congressional resolution on the Day of Silence in 2002 (GLSEN, 2011b, para. 8). That same year, Governor Gray Davis of California proclaimed the National Day of Silence as an official date, while more than 100,000 student activists participated in the protest nationwide (GLSEN, 2011b, para. 8). The event continues to swell, with the latest report from 2008 estimating student participation in the "hundreds of thousands" at over 8,000 schools worldwide (GLSEN, 2011b, para. 9).

It was no accident that an academic paper written by a young woman developed into an international protest drawing congressional support. The organizational materials are the product of years of rhetorical refinement. They include the yearly "Day of Silence Organizing Manual" with attendant materials for the event (i.e., recruiting posters, fundraising ideas, pamphlets, and guides for creating "safe places"). These materials are available on the National Day of Silence's website along with information on the event's history, legal status, and a list of organizations who have endorsed the Day of Silence. The materials allow local groups to personalize their event, although the national organizers have a vested interest in encoding a consistent and coherent message across the various local performances of the Day of Silence. Such consistency and coherence emerges from the organizing materials available to participants made available annually in an "organizing manual," which serves as a handbook on the rhetoric of social protest for participants.

Three interconnected features of the Day of Silence are particularly important for fostering a type of community capable of improving and then sustaining the health of LGBT youths. First, the organizing materials provide comprehensive information concerning the plight of LGBT communities, the legal rights and obligations of participants in the event, and details how to sustain pro-LGBT rights movements that utilize direct action organizing or single-issue campaigns. Second, the organizers actively embrace the diversity of participants. Rather than attempting to implement top-down control over a specific political agenda, the national project organizers provide direction for local individuals and groups to organize their own contributions to the event. The 2003 manual, which is the earliest manual archived after the merge with GLSEN, for instance, directed local organizers to select one local problem that they have the potential to change, which is a key tenet of direct action organizing (GLSEN, 2002, p. 11).

The most recent available organizing manual made available online to local organizers similarly indicates that the goal is to sustain a "voice" beyond the nine-hour event (GLSEN, 2011a). The third feature of the manual is the national organizers' focus on one element of the event: visibility. They see this visibility to be necessary for countering the institutional silencing of LGBT people and their allies. LGBT concerns are to become visible by disrupting norms of participation in daily life. "Silence" is then used as a rhetorical tactic that stands as demonstrative evidence of the effects of victimizing silencing that target LGBT people.

The organizing manual thus helps local organizers with general issues concerning activism and specific questions concerning the use of "silence" in the event. The lessons of the manual are put into action in the ancillary materials available to local organizers for use before and during their Day of Silence. The materials are designed to carry out three interconnected tasks: recruit participants, draw publicity, and encode meaning into the protest. Although local groups are directed to set their own goals, the national organizers proactively seek to control the use of these materials as they frame the protest. In using the materials, site organizers are subject to a "Resource Usage Agreement," stating that they agree to not use the materials "in a manner contrary to the spirit and goals of the Day of Silence" (GLSEN, 2007, para. 2).

A concise statement outlining the event's "spirit and goals" is presented on the "speaking cards" distributed by participants on the day of the event. The written text on the "speaking card" voices the protestor's reasons for being silent. In addition to being the primary means of communicating during the event, the organizers boast these cards as the "most captivating publicity tool [for the Day of Silence], because they are handed directly to individuals, and they provide the greatest opportunity for educating your school community" (GLSEN, 2002, p. 27). The text on the front side appears on many of the ancillary materials, including all of the ones discussed in this essay. The national organizers have changed the card's content over the years, though the text is not designed to be altered by local groups. These cards are consequently the most prominent medium used to disseminate the national organizers' message.

The front of the card contains a standard message concerning the event. The refinements from 2000 to 2011 indicate the national organizers' attention to rhetoric. The front of the "speaking card" used prior to 2002 read:

> Please understand my reasons for not speaking today. I support lesbian, gay, bisexual, and transgender rights. People who are silent today believe that laws and attitudes should be inclusive of people of all sexual orientations. The Day of Silence is to draw attention to those who have been silenced by hatred, oppression, and prejudice. Think about the voices you are not hearing. What can you do to end the silence? (Day of Silence Project, 1999, para. 1).

This early version claims that the event memorializes "silence" as inequality and prejudice. The goal of the protest is to draw attention to those (the people) silenced. The cards lack the reasoning for readers to accept the protestors' "belief" that laws and attitudes must be revised to reflect social equality. This leaves the grounds for achieving the protest's goals couched in the language of personal belief rather than justice. The shaky grounds are further weakened by the call for reflection rather than action in the last two sentences. The readers are first asked to contemplate silence in general, and second consider their capabilities for acting to end the silence. Given the framing, this call for action is designed to draw a productive response primarily from people who are already disposed favorably towards LGBT rights.

The national organizers revised the "speaking cards" after partnering with GLSEN. The revisions addressed the earlier version's shortcomings and shifted the focus from the rhetoric of social equality to that of a struggle against injustice. It reads:

> Please understand my reasons for not speaking today. I am participating in the Day of Silence, a national youth movement protesting the silence faced by lesbian, gay, bisexual and transgender people and their allies. My deliberate silence echoes that silence, which is caused by harassment, prejudice, and discrimination. I believe that enduring the silence is the first step towards fighting these injustices. Think about the voices you are not

hearing today. What are you going to do to end the silence? (GLSEN, 2003, para. 1).

In this locution, the explicit goal is to fight against the injustices of anti-LGBT harassment, prejudice, and discrimination. "Silence" is a deliberate rhetorical tactic *endured* to make visible the harm of anti-LGBT oppression. Like the earlier version, the last two sentences challenge the readers to act, though the challenges are clearly more insistent in this version. The readers are first instructed to contemplate the silence that they are bearing witness to during the event, and second are asked to become part of the solution for ending the silence.

The speaking cards have been further refined to focus on explicitly confronting systemic victimization. It reads:

> Please understand my reasons for not speaking today. I am participating in the Day of Silence (DOS), a national youth movement bringing attention to the silence faced by lesbian, gay, bisexual and transgender people and their allies. My deliberate silence echoes that silence, which is caused by anti-LGBT bullying, name-calling and harassment. I believe that ending the silence is the first step towards building awareness and making a commitment to address these injustices. Think about the voices you are not hearing today. What are you going to do to end the silence? (GLSEN, 2011a, p. 20).

"Silence" is no longer something to be endured but rather the external manifestation of systemic injustices that are to be ended. Mirroring the research about behaviors that cause negative health consequences for LGBT people, the focus has shifted to confronting concrete problems, including bullying, name-calling, and harassment. As such, the rhetorical design of the most recent "speaking cards" challenge people to combat the root causes of anti-LGBT discrimination.

LIMITATIONS

Joan Wallach Scott argues, "[m]aking visible the experience of a different group exposes the existence of repressive mechanisms, but not their inner workings or logics; we know that difference exists, but we don't understand it as constituted relationally" (1992, p. 25). In accounting for several manifestations of silence used by, for, and against LGBT communities, the multiple repressive forces emerged as "interested act[s] of power or domination" (Scott, p. 25). These various acts were performed in hopes of reconstituting subjects through experiencing particular forms of "silence." Rhetorical analysis demonstrates the inner workings or logics of these rhetorical deployments of "silence" by hate crimes, suicides, and myriad health consequences that are promoted by systemic anti-LGBT discrimination.

Those political activists who emerged in response to Gunn's death and those who join together in silence to challenge a broad spectrum of injustices targeting LGBT people indicate how silence can simultaneously serve as a resource for promoting health. As Foucault (1990) argued, silence does not signify the absolute limit of discourse but rather is an integral part of language and action. As such, we have witnessed many silences that, for better or worse, emerge as powerful rhetorical tactics. Just as silence can kill and make sick, so too, it can be harnessed, like it was by those 2,500 youths in Newark and by hundreds of thousands of people over the years during National Day of Silence events.

In order to gain a more comprehensive view of political activism as a health-giving activity, it is necessary to conduct research on individual movements, their effects on LGBT health, and cultural norms toward LGBT people and issues. This includes ad hoc movements that emerge on the coattails of horrific violence and longstanding movements that have worked over time to fight for LGBT people. As a better understanding of the negative health consequences of discrimination and positive health consequences of certain forms of political activism emerges, it is important to identify those practices most useful for pro-LGBT advocacy.

NOTE

1. Kim Pearson provides comparative data between major news coverage of the murders of Matthew Shepard and all news for Sakia Gunn. In the month that the events occurred, Shepard's story was covered 448 times, whereas Gunn was covered eight times. In the first eleven months, there were a total of 735 stories about Shepard and twenty-eight about Gunn (Pearson, 2006, p. 169).

Appendix A

INTERVIEW QUESTIONS

Demographic Questions

1. How do you identify, in terms of gender?
2. What pronouns do you prefer?
3. How old are you?
4. What is the highest level of education you have achieved?
5. In what state do you currently live?
6. Where have you lived? For how long?
7. What is your occupation or profession? How long have you held this position?
8. Do you consider yourself religious or spiritual, or do you identify with any religious affiliation?
9. How would you identify yourself in terms of culture or ethnicity?
10. How much would you estimate as your annual income?

Transgender Status and Transition

11. When, and how, did you know that you were transgender?
12. What led up to your decision to transition?
    a. What factors, if any, inhibited your decision to transition? (what people would think, fears about societal reactions . . .)
    b. What factors, if any, encouraged or facilitated your decision to transition?
13. How far are you into your transition? (hormones, top surgery, bottom surgery, etc.)

14. How long ago did you start passing as your preferred gender?
15. How did you transition in the realms of your life (family, friends, community, etc.)?
16. What types of negative reactions have you encountered when disclosing your gender identity?
17. What types of positive reactions have you encountered when disclosing your gender identity?

Experiences with Health Professionals

18. Growing up, how would you describe your experiences with doctors?
19. How would you describe your health right now? How would you describe your health overall?
20. Describe the ideal relationship you would like to have with your doctor. To what extent is this similar (or different) from the relationship you have now?
21. Did you see the same general doctor after transition as you did before transition?
22. How often have you been to the doctor since you started identifying as your preferred gender?
23. Can you describe instances where you had experiences that prevented adequate treatment when visiting the doctor?
24. How has your identity, or the way you view yourself, changed since your visits with your doctor?
25. What differences have you noted in your doctor's behavior pre- and post-transition?
26. What behavior changes have you noticed in yourself with visiting the doctor pre- and post-transition?
27. How do doctors tend to communicate with you? (medical jargon, everyday terms, etc.)
28. Each person holds several identities: work identity, social identity, personal identity, health identity. That being said, how would you describe your health identity? [Prepared elaboration on health identity: our identity in terms of our health or a medical issue.]
29. How have your doctor's visits impacted your health identity, if they have at all?

Appendix B

$\mathcal{W}$e chose not to include a chart specifying the demographics of each participant due to the small sample sizes (n = 40, n = 21) and risks associated with a breach in participant confidentiality. Overall sample characteristics and noteworthy trends are bulleted below.

Sex Assigned at Birth and Gender Identity

- Slightly less than half of participants were sexed male at birth (n = 27) than those sexed female at birth (n = 33). One participant was sexed female at birth and reclassified as male at three months of age. This individual is coded as intersex (n = 1).
- For self-identified sex and gender, the participants fell into five main categories: Woman/Female-Only (n=11); Man/Male-Only (n=9); Woman/Female and Trans (n=11); Man/Male and Trans (n=13); and, Genderqueer (n=15). Additionally, one person identified as a male-to-female transsexual genderqueer, and another identified as bigender.
- There are those who assert a binary and nontrans classification (n=20) and those who identify with some type of trans or nonbinary classification (n=41).

Age, Race, Sexuality, and Relationship Status

- In Kelly's sample, the average age of participants was thirty-six years old, with a range of twenty to seventy years of age. Participants sexed male at birth had a larger age range (twenty-one to seventy years) and a higher mean (forty years) than those sexed female at birth (range: twenty to fifty-three years; mean: thirty-one years).

- In Nordmarken's sample, the average age of participants was forty years old, ranging from twenty to sixty-one years of age.
- In Kelly's sample, the largest self-reported racial and ethnic group in the sample was white, Caucasian, or European (n=24, 60 percent), followed by black or African American (n=4, 10 percent), white and Native American/American Indian (n=4, 10 percent), Hispanic or Latino only (n=3, 7.5 percent); and, white and Hispanic or Latino (n=2, 5 percent). One person each reported the following racial and ethnic identities: Arabic; black, Native American, and white; and, South Asian.
- In Nordmarken's sample, the largest self-reported racial and ethnic group in the sample was white (n=12). The other reported racial and ethnic identities consisted of "light skinned" African American (n=1), "of African descent" (n=1), Thai (n=1), Native American (n=1), and Japanese/Asian American (n=1). Multiethnic/multiracial identities reported were Thai/white (n=1), Cherokee/Korean (n=1), Cherokee/white (n=1), Spanish/olive-skinned/white (n=1).
- In Kelly's sample, the most common terms that individuals used to identify their sexuality was straight or heterosexual (n=8), bisexual (n=7), queer (n=7), and pansexual or polysexual (n=5). Quite a few rejected identity labels altogether (n=5), two identified as asexual, two more identified as gay, and the rest described their sexuality in terms of an "attraction to women" (n=3) or an "attraction to men" (n=1). Nordmarken did not systematically collect data on sexuality.
- In Kelly's sample, almost half of the participants identified their relationship status as single (n=19), three of which were in the process of a divorce. Half of the participants reported a formal coupling as married (n=5), in a domestic partnership (n=1), engaged (n=3), in a life partnership (n=3), or in a relationship (n=8). In addition, one individual identified their relationship status as being a member of a polyamorous family. Nordmarken did not collect data on relationship status.

Educational Attainment and Occupation

- In Kelly and Nordmarken's combined data, all participants had completed high school, approximately one-third enrolled in college but did not hold a degree (n=22), another third held an associate's (n=3) or bachelor's (n=15) degree (one of which also held a teaching credential), and the last third held advanced degrees (Master's, n=11; PhD, n=5; JD, n=2).
- Just over half of the participants had semiskilled to professional occupations in the fields of education (n=2), academia (n=2), arts and

entertainment (n=4), health and human services (n=6), civil service (n=2), security (n=2), technology and engineering (n=7), hardware contracting (n=1), law (n=2), administration (n=1), and program management (n=2). A small group of individuals worked in reportedly lower-paying, semiskilled occupations (retail, n=4; custodial, n=1; customer service, n=2; nanny, n=1; delivery driver, n=1; carpentry, n=1; fundraiser, n=1).

- Approximately 30 percent of the sample did not have full-time employment, and of this group two received veteran's benefits, another two received disability benefits, and nine individuals defined their occupational status as a full-time student.

Residence, Veteran's Status and Disability

- Twenty-seven of the participants claimed residence in a large city, whereas the rest were spread out across the suburbs (n=7), in small towns and/or rural locations (n=10), and in small- to medium-sized cities (n=17). Four individuals were temporarily residing in the United States since they were not U.S. citizens.
- Four participants were military veterans, and two identified as disabled and were receiving disability benefits as their primary source of income. It is possible that more individuals in the sample were veterans and/ or disabled. There were no direct questions about these characteristics.

Hormone and Surgical Status

- Nordmarken did not collect hormone- and surgery-related data for all of his respondents, but of the data collected, eight had no hormones and no surgery, four had hormones and no surgery, and five had hormones and surgery, with at least two having had genital surgery (missing data for three respondents).★
- In Kelly's sample, 30 percent of participants were not on hormones, and had no surgery; 42 percent were on hormones, with no surgeries; 28 percent were on hormones and postoperative (15 percent had genital surgery). The group of "hormones and surgery" was oversampled for the purposes of having a more even distribution across these three categories.
- Seventy percent of the participants (n=28) were on hormone replacement therapy ranging from a period of six months to twenty-one years. The use of hormones was fairly even across sex assigned at birth (male, n=14; female, n=13; intersex, n=1), as was the absence of hormone use (male, n=6; female n=6).

- The breakdown of genital surgery and chest surgery across sex assigned at birth is as follows: vaginoplasty (male, n=2; intersex, n=1); orchiectomy only (male, n=1); metoidioplasty (female, n=2); chest surgery (female, n=8; male, n=1; intersex, n=1).
- Of the twenty-nine who did not have surgery, eight identified explicitly as "non-op" or having no current interest in surgery, one individual was weeks away from undergoing SRS, and twelve expressed an explicit desire for surgery. The rest reported mixed feelings about surgery, stating interest but also expressing fear of surgery in general, the lack of insurance coverage, or displeasure with the potential results.
- The group of individuals in the "hormones and surgery" group were less likely to be white (40 percent) and more likely to reside in a big city (45 percent) than those in the overall sample (60 percent white, 15 percent big city).
- Individuals in the "hormones, no surgery" group were more likely to be white (69 percent) than those in the overall sample (60 percent white) and less likely to live in a big city (6 percent).

Documented Identity

- Although 70 percent of the sample had undergone body alterations through hormones and/or surgery at the time of the interview, only half made any changes to the sex marker on their primary identity documents.
- Of the twenty individuals who made changes to their identity documents half (n=10) reclassified the sex on their driver's license only. Only 18 percent of the individuals in the sample reclassified the sex on their birth certificate (n=7), four of whom also reclassified the sex on their passport.

NOTE

*Nordmarken did not collect hormone, surgery, and documented legal identity related data for all of his respondents, so the sample characteristics percentages on hormone, surgical status, and documented identity describe Kelly's sample.

Bibliography

2012 National Health Care Disparities Report. (2013). Retrieved from http://www
.ahrq.gov/research/findings/nhqrdr/nhdr12/index.html.

Abbott, J., Johnson, R., Koziol-McLain, J., & Lowenstein, S. R. (1995). Domestic
violence against women. *JAMA: The Journal of the American Medical Association,*
273(22), 1763–1767.

Adams, M. L. (1989). You're all right so long as you act nice: Lesbians' experience of
the North American health system. *Fireweed, 28,* 53–67.

Adams, T. E. (2011). *Narrating the closet: An autoethnography of same-sex attraction.* Wal-
nut Creek, CA: Left Coast.

Allen, B. J. (2004). *Difference matters: Communicating social identity.* (2nd ed.). Long
Grove, IL: Waveland Press.

Almeida, J., Johnson, R. M., Corliss, H. L., Molnar, B. E., & Azrael, D. (2009). Emotional distress among LGBT youth: The influence of perceived discrimination on
sexual orientation. *Journal of Youth Adolescence, 38*(7), 1001–1014.

Alpert, E. J. (1995). Violence in intimate relationships and the practicing internist: new
"disease," or new agenda? *Annals of Internal Medicine, 123*(10), 774–781.

Amadio, D. (2006). Internalized homophobia, alcohol use, and alcohol-related problems among lesbian and gay men. *Addictive Behaviors, 31*(7), 1153–1162.

Ambert, A. M., Adler, P. A., Adler, P., & Detzner, D. F. (1995). Understanding and
evaluating qualitative research. *Journal of Marriage and the Family, 57*(4), 879–893.

American Medical Association. (2004). *Code of ethics: Opinion 2.05—Artificial insemi-*
nation by anonymous donor. Retrieved from http://www.ama-assn.org//ama/pub/
physician-resources/medical-ethics/code-medical-ethics/opinion205.page.

American Psychiatric Association. (2000). *Diagnostic and statistical manual of mental dis-*
orders (4th ed.). Washington, DC: American Psychiatric Association.

American Psychiatric Association. (2013). *Diagnostic and statistical manual of mental*
disorders (5th ed.). http://dx.doi.org/10.1176/appi.books.9780890425596.910646.

Angrosino, M. V. (2005). Recontextualizing observation: Ethnography, pedagogy,
and the prospects for a progressive political agenda. *The Sage handbook of qualitative*
research, 3, 729–745.

Aramburu Alegria, C. (2011). Transgender identity and health care: Implications for psychosocial and physical evaluation. *Journal of the American Academy of Nurse Practitioners, 23,* 175–182.

Ard, K., & Makadon, H. (2013). Improving the healthcare of lesbian, gay, bisexual, and transgender people: Understanding and eliminating health disparities. *The National LGBT Health Education Center, Fenway Institute.* Retrieved from http://www.lgbthealtheducation.org/.

Arons, J. (2007). *Future choices: Assisted reproductive technologies and the law.* Retrieved from http://www.americanprogress.org/issues/women/report/2007/12/17/3728/future-choices-assisted-reproductive-technologies-and-the-law/.

Ash, M. A., & Badgett, M. V. L. (2006). Separate and unequal: The effect of unequal access to employment-based health insurance on gay, lesbian, and bisexual people. *Contemporary Economic Policy, 24*(4), 582–599.

Bacon, J. (1998). Getting the story straight: Coming out narratives and the possibility of a cultural rhetoric. *World Englishes, 17*(2), 249–258.

Badgett, M. V. L. (2007). *Unequal taxes on equal benefits: The taxation of domestic partner benefits. The Williams Institute.* Retrieved from http://williamsinstitute.law.ucla.edu/wp-content/uploads/Badgett-UnequalTaxesOnEqualBenefits-Dec-2007.pdf.

Badgett, M. V. L. (2010). The economic value of marriage for same-sex couples. *Drake Law Review, 58*(4), 1081–1116.

Baker, K. (2012, November 27). Ending gay and transgender health disparities. *Center for American Progress.* Retrieved from http://www.americanprogress.org/issues/lgbt/news/2012/11/27/46035/ending-gay-and-transgender-health-disparities/.

Balsam, K. F. (2001). Nowhere to hide: Lesbian battering, homophobia, and minority stress. *Women & Therapy, 23*(3), 25–37.

Balsam, K. F., & Szymanski, D. M. (2005). Relationship quality and domestic violence in women's same-sex relationships: The role of minority stress. *Psychology of Women Quarterly, 29*(3), 258–269.

Balsam, K. F., Molina, Y., Beadnell, B., Simoni, J., & Walters, K. (2011). Measuring multiple minority stress: The LGBT people of color microaggressions scale. *Cultural Diversity and Ethnic Minority Psychology, 17*(2), 163–174.

Bates, N., DeMaio, T. J., Robins, C., & Hicks, W. (2012). *Classifying relationship and marital status among same-sex couples* (Research Report Series #2012–01). Washington, DC: U.S. Census Bureau. Retrieved from http://www.census.gov/srd/papers/pdf/rsm2012-01.pdf.

Baum, A., Garofalo, J. P., & Yali, A. M. (2006). Socioeconomic status and chronic stress: Does stress account for SES effects on health? *Annals of the New York Academy of Sciences, in Socioeconomic Status and Health in Industrial Nations: Social, Psychological, and Biological Pathways, 896,* 131–144.

Baxter, L. A. (2004). Relationships as dialogues. *Personal Relationships, 11*(1), 1–22.

Baxter, L. A. (2011). *Voicing relationships: A dialogic perspective.* Thousand Oaks, CA: Sage.

Bayer, R. (1987). *Homosexuality and American psychiatry: The politics of diagnosis* (2nd Ed.). Princeton, NJ: Princeton University Press.

Becker, G., Gates, R. J., & Newsom, E. (2004). Self-care among chronically ill African-Americans: Culture, health disparities, and health insurance status. *American Journal of Public Health, 94*(12), 2006–2073.

Beemyn, G., & Rankin, S. (2011). *The lives of transgender people.* Chichester, NY: Columbia University Press.

Berger, R. M. (1996). *Gay and gray: The older homosexual man* (2nd Ed.). Binghamton, NY: Harrington Park Press.

Billings, D. B., & Urban, T. (1982). The socio-medical construction of transsexualism: An interpretation and critique. *Social Problems, 29,* 266–282.

Black, D. A., Sanders, S. F., & Taylor, L. J. (2007). The economics of lesbian and gay families. *Journal of Economic Perspectives, 21*(2), 53–70.

Blosnich, J. R., & Bossarte, R. M. (2009). Comparisons of intimate partner violence among partners in same-sex and opposite-sex relationships in the United States. *American Journal of Public Health, 99*(12), 2182–2184.

Bockting, W. O., Robinson, B., Benner, A., & Scheltema, K. (2010). Patient satisfaction with transgender health services. *Journal of Sex and Marital Therapy, 30*(4), 277–294. doi: 10.1080/00926230490422467.

Boehmer, U. (2002). Twenty years of public health research: Inclusion of lesbian, gay, bisexual, and transgender populations. *American Journal of Public Health, 92*(7), 1125–1130.

Boehmer, U., & Bowen, D. J. (2009). Examining factors linked to overweight and obesity in women of different sexual orientations. *Preventive Medicine, 48,* 357–361.

Boehmer, U., Bowen, D. J., & Bauer, G. R. (2007). Overweight and obesity in sexual-minority women: Evidence from population-based data. *American Journal of Public Health, 97*(6), 1134–1140.

Bond, L., Carlin, J. B., Thomas, L., Rubin, K., & Patton, G. (2001). Does bullying cause emotional problems? A prospective study of young teenagers. *British Medical Journal, 323*(7311), 480–484.

Bontempo, D. E., & D'Augelli, A. R. (2002). Effects of at-school victimization and sexual orientation on lesbian, gay, or bisexual youths' health risk behavior. *Society for Adolescent Medicine, 30*(5), 364–374.

Bossarte, R. M., Swahn, M. H., & Breiding, M. (2009). Racial, ethnic, and sex differences in the associations between violence and self-reported health among US high school students. *Journal of School Health, 79*(2), 74–81.

Bradford, J., Ryan, C., & Rothblum E. D. (1994). National lesbian health care survey. *Journal of Consulting and Clinical Psychology, 62*(2), 228–242.

Branham R. J., & W. Pearce, B. (1985). Between text and context: Toward a rhetoric of contextual reconstruction. *Quarterly Journal of Speech, 71*(1), 19–36.

Braun, V., & Clarke, V. (2006). Using thematic analysis in psychology. *Qualitative Research in Psychology, 3*(2), 77–101.

Breiding, M. J., Black, M. C., & Ryan, G. W. (2008). Chronic disease and health risk behaviors associated with intimate partner violence, 18 U.S. states/territories, 2005. *Annals of Epidemiology, 18*(7), 538–544.

Brown, J. B., Stewart, M. A., & Ryan, B. L. (2003). Outcomes of patient-provider interaction. In T. L. Thompson, A. M. Dorsey, K. I. Miller, & R. Parrot (Eds.), *Handbook of health communication* (pp. 141–161). Mahwah, NJ: Lawrence Erlbaum.

Brummett, B. (1984). Rhetorical theory as heuristic and moral: A pedagogical justification. *Communication Education, 33*(2), 91–107.

Buchmueller, T., & Carpenter, C. (2010). Disparities in health insurance coverage, access, and outcomes for individuals in same-sex versus different-sex relationships, 2000–2007. *American Journal of Public Health, 100*(3), 489–495.

Budge, S. L., Adelson, J. L., & Howard, K. A. S. (2013, February 11). Anxiety and depression in transgender individuals: The roles of transition status, loss, social support, and coping. *Journal of Consulting and Clinical Psychology.* Advance online publication. doi: 10.1037/a0031774.

Bundesärztekammer. (2009). Richtlinien über künstliche Befruchtung. *Bundesanzeiger 145*(3), 373.

Bundesministerium für Familie, Senioren, Frauen und Jugend. (2013). *Adoption: Voraussetzungen für die Adoption eines minderjährigen Kindes.* Retrieved from http://www.familien-wegweiser.de/wegweiser/stichwortverzeichnis,did=101188.html.

Burke, T. W., Jordan, M. L., & Owen, S. S. (2002). A cross-national comparison of gay and lesbian domestic violence. *Journal of Contemporary Criminal Justice, 18*(3), 231–257.

Burroway, Jim. (2008). *In Box Turtle Bulletin.*

Burton, C. M., Marshal, M. P., Chisolm, D. J., Sucato, G. S., & Friedman, M. S. (2013). Sexual minority-related victimization as a mediator of mental health disparities in sexual minority youth: A longitudinal analysis. *Journal of Youth and Adolescence, 42/3*(394–402), 0047–2891.

Calasanti, T. M., & Slevin, K. F. (2001). *Gender, social inequalities, and aging.* Gender Lens Series. Lanham, MD: Alta Mira Press.

Campbell, J. C. (2002). Health consequences of intimate partner violence. *The Lancet, 359*(9314), 1331–1336.

Campbell, R., & Wasco, S. M. (2005). Understanding rape and sexual assault: 20 years of progress and future directions. *Journal of Interpersonal Violence, 20*(1), 127–131.

Carpenter, C., & Gates, G. J. (2008). Gay and lesbian partnership: Evidence from California. *Demography, 45*(3), 573–590.

Case Western Reserve University. (2013). *Coming Out.* Retrieved from http://case.edu/lgbt/safezone/comingout.html.

Cass, V. C. (1979). Homosexual identity formation: A theoretical model. *Journal of Homosexuality, 4*(3), 219–235.

Cass, V. C. (1984). Homosexual identity: A concept in need of a definition. *Journal of Homosexuality, 9*(2/3), 105–126.

Castle Bell, G. (2012). "I still have a dream . . .": Exploring black and white communication challenges in 21st century United States (Doctoral dissertation). Retrieved from ProQuest database (10079).

Caughlin, J. P., Koerner, A. F., Schrodt, P., & Fitzpatrick, M. A. (2011). Interpersonal communication in family relationships. In M. L. Knapp & J. A. Daly (Eds.), *The*

Sage handbook of interpersonal communication (4th ed.) (pp. 679–714). Thousand Oaks, CA: Sage.

Centers for Disease Control. (2010). *Web-based injury statistics query and reporting system.* Retrieved from http://www.cdc.gov/injury/wisqars/.

Centers for Disease Control. (2011). Sexual identity, sex of sexual contacts, and health-risk behaviors among students in grades 9–12: Youth risk behavior surveillance, selected sites, United States, 2001–2009. *Morbidity and Mortality Weekly Report Surveillance Summaries, 60*(7), 1–133.

Centers for Disease Control. (2012). *About the U.S. ART clinic reporting system.* Retrieved from http://www.cdc.gov/art/ART2010/faq.htm#6.

Chan, C. S. (1989). Issues of identity development among Asian-American lesbians and gay men. *Journal of Counseling and Development, 68*(1), 18–20.

Chan, C. S. (1995). Issues of sexual identity in an ethnic minority: The case of Chinese American lesbians, gay men, and bisexual people. In A. R. D'Augelli & C. J. Patterson, (Eds.), *Lesbian, gay, and bisexual identities over the lifespan: Psychological perspectives* (pp. 87–101). New York: Oxford University.

Chirrey, D. A. (2003). I hereby come out: What sort of speech act is coming out? *Journal of Sociolinguistics, 7*(1), 24–37.

Christians, C. G., & Carey, J. W. (1989). The logic and aims of qualitative research. In G. H. I. Stempel & B. H. Westley (Eds.), *Research methods in mass communication* (pp. 354–374). Englewood Cliffs, NJ: Prentice Hall.

Cianciotto, J., & Cahill, S. (2003). *Education policy: Issues affecting lesbian, gay, bisexual, and transgender youth.* Washington, DC: National Gay and Lesbian Task Force Policy Institute.

Claxton, G., Rae, M., Panchel, N., Damico, A., Lundy, J., Bostick, N., Kenward, K., & Whitmore, H. (2012). *Employer health benefits 2012 annual survey* (#8345). Retrieved from http://kff.org/health-costs/report/employer-health-benefits-2012-annual-survey/.

Clifford, D., Hertz, F., & Doskow, E. (2012). *A legal guide for lesbian and gay couples.* San Francisco: NOLO.

Cochran, S. D., & Mays, V. M. (1988). Disclosure of sexual preference to physicians by black lesbian and bisexual women. *The Western Journal of Medicine, 149*(5), 616–619.

Cochran, S. D., & Mays, V. M. (2006). Physical health complaints among lesbian, gay men, and bisexual and homosexually experienced heterosexual individuals: Results from the California Quality of Life Survey. *American Journal of Public Health, 9*(11), 2048–2055.

Cochran, S. D., Mays, V. M., Alegria, M., Ortega, A. N., & Takeuchi, D. (2007). Mental health and substance use disorders among Latino and Asian American lesbian, gay, and bisexual adults. *Journal of Consulting and Clinical Psychology, 75*(5). 785–794.

Cohen, R. A., Makuc, D. M., Bernstein, A. B., Bilheimer, L. T., & Powell-Griner, E. (2009). *Health insurance coverage trends, 1959–2007: Estimates from the national health interview survey* (No. 17). Hyattsville, MD: National Center for Health Statistics. Retrieved from http://www.cdc.gov/nchs/data/nhsr/nhsr017.pdf.

Coker, A. L., Davis, K. E., Arias, I., Desai, S., Sanderson, M., Brandt, H. M., et al. (2002). Physical and mental health effects of intimate partner violence for men and women. *American Journal of Preventive Medicine, 23*(4), 260–268.

Coker, A. L., Smith, P. H., Thompson, M. P., McKeown, R. E., Bethea, L., & Davis, K. E. (2002). Social support protects against the negative effects of partner violence on mental health. *Journal of Women's Health & Gender-Based Medicine, 11*(5), 465–476.

Coleman, E., et al. (2011). Standards of care for the health of transsexual, transgender, and gender-nonconforming people, Version 7. *International Journal of Transgenderism,* 13: 165–232.

Collins, P. H. (1986). Learning from the outsider within: The sociological significance of black feminist thought. *Social Problems, 33*(6), S14–S32.

Coston, B. (2011). *Issues in intimate violence: Heterosexism and exclusion.* Oxford: Peter Lang Publishing.

Cowan, R. S. (1983). *More work for mother: The ironies of household technology from the open hearth to the microwave.* Basic Books, Inc.

Cox, N., Dewaele, A., Van Houtte, M., & Vincke, J. (2011). Stress-related growth, coming out, and internalized homonegativity in lesbian, gay, and bisexual youth: An examination of stress-related growth within the minority stress model. *Journal of Homosexuality, 58*(1), 117–137.

Cramer, D. W., & Roach, A. J. (1988). Coming out to mom and dad: A study of gay males and their relationships with their parents. *Journal of Homosexuality, 15*(3–4), 79–91.

Cramer, R. J., McNiel, D. E., Holley, S. R., Shumway, M., & Boccellari, A. (2012). Mental health in violent crime victims: Does orientation matter? *Law and Human Behavior, 36*(2), 87–95.

Cray, A., & Baker, K. (2012, October 3). FAQ: Health insurance needs for transgenderAmericans. *Center for American Progress.* Retrieved from http://www.americanprogress.org/issues/lgbt/report/2012/10/03/40334/faq-health-insurance-needs-for-transgender-americans/.

Cray, A., & Baker, K. (2013, May 30). How the Affordable Care Act helps the LGBT community. *Center for American Progress.* Retrieved from http://www.americanprogress.org/issues/lgbt/news/2013/05/30/64609/how-the-affordable-care-act-helps-the-lgbt-community/.

Creswell, J. W. (2009). *Research design: Qualitative, quantitative, and mixed methods approaches* (3rd ed.). Thousand Oaks, CA: Sage.

Crimmel, B. L. (2011). *Self-insured coverage in employer-sponsored health insurance for the private sector, 2000 and 2010* (Statistical Brief 339). Retrieved from http://meps.ahrq.gov/data_files/publications/st339/stat339.pdf.

Cromwell, J. (1999). *Transmen and FTMs: Identities, bodies, genders, and sexuality.* Urbana: University of Illinois Press.

Croteau, J. (1996). Research on the work experiences of lesbian, gay, and bisexual people: An integrative review of methodology and findings. *Journal of Vocational Behavior, 48*(2), 195–209.

Cruikshank, M. (2009). *Learning to be old: Gender, culture, and aging.* New York: Rowman & Littlefield Publishers.

D'Augelli, A. R. (1994). Identity development and sexual orientation: Toward a model of lesbian, gay, and bisexual development. In E. J. Trickett, R. J. Watts, &

D. Birman, (Eds.), *Human diversity: Perspectives on people in context* (pp. 312–333). San Francisco: Jossey-Bass.

D'Augelli, A. R., Grossman, A. H., Salter, N. P., Vasey, J. J., Starks, M. T., & Sinclair, K. O. (2005). Predicting the suicide attempts of lesbian, gay, and bisexual youth. *Suicide and Life Threatening Behavior, 35*(6), 646–660.

D'Augelli, A. R., Grossman, A. H., & Starks, M. T. (2006). Childhood gender atypicality, victimization, and PTSD among lesbian, gay, and bisexual youth. *Journal of Interpersonal Violence, 21*(11), 1462–1482.

Day of Silence Project (1999). *The Day of Silence Project.* Retreived from http://web.archive.org/web/19990421121847/http://www.youth-guard.org/dayofsilence/index.html.

Dean, L., Meyer, I. H., Robinson, K., Sell, R. L., Sember, R., Silenzio, V. M., et al. (2000). Lesbian, gay, bisexual, and transgender health: Findings and concerns. *Journal of the Gay and Lesbian Medical Association, 4*(3), 102–151.

DeBold, K. (2007). Focus on lesbian health. *The Women's Health Activist,* March/April, 1–7.

Defense of Marriage Act, Pub. L. 104–199, 1 USC §7 and 28 USC §1738C (1996).

Denzin, N. K., & Lincoln, Y. S. (2011). *The Sage handbook of qualitative research.* Thousand Oaks, CA: Sage.

Dewey, J. M. (2008). Knowledge legitimacy: How trans-patient behavior supports and challenges current medical knowledge. *Qualitative Health Research, 18*(10), 1345–1355. doi: 10.177/1049732308324247.

Diamond, L. M. (2003). Was it a phase? Young women's relinquishment of lesbian/bisexual identities over a 5–year period. *Journal of Personality and Social Psychology, 84*(2), 352–364.

Diaz, R. M., Ayala, G., Bein, E., Henne, J., & Marin, B.V. (2001). The impact of homophobia, poverty, and racism on the mental health of gay and bisexual Latino men: Findings in 3 US Cities. *American Journal of Public Health, 9*(6), 927–932.

Dibble, S. L., Roberts, S. A., Robertson, P. A., & Paul, S. M. (2002). Risk factors for ovarian cancer: Lesbian and heterosexual women [Online Exclusive]. *Oncology Nursing Forum, 29*(1), E1–E7.

Dienemann, J., Boyle, E., Baker, D., Resnick, W., Wiederhorn, N., & Campbell, J. (2000). Intimate partner abuse among women diagnosed with depression. *Issues in Mental Health Nursing, 21*(5), 499–513.

Diep, F. (2013, July 15). More U.S. hospitals now guarantee equal care for gay patients. *Popular Science.* Retrieved from http://www.popsci.com/science/article/2013–07/more-us-hospitals-now-guarantee-equal-care-gay-patients.

Dilley, J. A., Simmons, K. W., Boysun, M. J., Pizacani, B. A., & Stark, M. J. (2010). Demonstrating the importance and feasibility of including sexual orientation in public health surveys: Health disparities in the Pacific Northwest. *American Journal of Public Health, 100*(3), 460–467.

Dobash, R. (1992). *Women, violence and social change.* London, England: Routledge.

Dolan, K. A., & Davis, P. W. (2003). Nuances and shifts in lesbian women's constructions of STI and HIV vulnerability. *Social Science & Medicine, 57*(1), 25–38.

Downs, A. (2005). *The velvet rage: Overcoming the pain of growing up gay in a straight man's world.* Cambridge, MA: Perseus Book Group.

Drescher, J. (1998). *Psychoanalytic therapy and the gay man.* Hillsdale, NJ: The Analytic Press.

du Pré, A. (2010). *Communicating about health: Current issues and perspectives* (3rd ed.). New York, NY: Oxford University Press.

Duberman, M. B., Vicinus, M., & Chauncey, Jr., G. (Eds.). (1989). *Hidden from history: Reclaiming the gay and lesbian past.* New York: New American Library.

Dutton, M. A., Green, B. L., Kaltman, S. I., Roesch, D. M., Zeffiro, T. A., & Krause, E. D. (2006). Intimate partner violence, PTSD, and adverse health outcomes. *Journal of Interpersonal Violence, 21*(7), 955–968.

Dwyer, S. C., & Buckle, J. L. (2009). The space between: On being an insider-outsider in qualitative research. *International Journal of Qualitative Methods, 8*(1), 54–63.

Eaklor, V. L. (2008). *Queer America: A GLBT history of the 20th century.* Westport, CT: Greenwood Press.

Egendorf, L. K. (2002). *An aging population: Opposing viewpoints.* San Diego, CA: Greenhaven Press.

Eguchi, S. (2009). Negotiation hegemonic masculinity: The rhetorical strategy of "straight-acting" among gay men. *Journal of Intercultural Communication Research, 38*(3), 193–209.

Eisenberg, M. E., & Aalsma, M. C. (2005). Bullying and peer victimization: Position paper of the Society for Adolescent Medicine. *Journal of Adolescent Health, 36*(1), 88–91.

Eliason, M. J., Dibble, S. L., Gordon, R., & Soliz, G. B. (2012). The Last Drag: an evaluation of an LGBT-specific smoking intervention. *Journal of Homosexuality, 59*(6), 864–878.

Eliason, M. J., & Schope, R. (2001). Does "don't ask don't tell" apply to health care? Lesbian, gay, and bisexual people's disclosure to health care providers. *Journal of the Gay and Lesbian Medical Association, 5*(4), 125–134.

Ellis, H. (1915). *Studies in the psychology of sex (3rd ed, 1936).* New York: Random House.

Ellsberg, M., Jansen, H. A. F. M., Heise, L., Watts, C. H., & Garcia-Moreno, C. (2008). Intimate partner violence and women's physical and mental health in the WHO multi-country study on women's health and domestic violence: an observational study. *The Lancet, 371*(9619), 1165–1172.

Epstein, D. (1999). Effective intervention in domestic violence cases: Rethinking the roles of prosecutors, judges, and the court system. *Yale Journal of Law & Feminism, 11*, 3–50.

Espelage, D. L., Aragon, S. R., Birkett, M., & Koenig, B. W. (2008). Homophobic teasing, psychological outcomes, and sexual orientation among high school students: What influence do parents and schools have? *School Psychology Review, 37*(2), 202–216.

Federal Bureau of Investigation. (2011). *Hate crime statistics 2011.* Retrieved from http://www.fbi.gov/about-us/cjis/ucr/hate-crime/2011/tables/table-1.

Feinleib, M. R. (Ed.). (1989). *Report of the secretary's task force on youth suicide. Volume 3: Prevention and interventions in youth suicide.* Rockville, MD: Alcohol, Drug Abuse, and Mental Health Administration.

Fischbach, R. L., & Herbert, B. (1997). Domestic violence and mental health: correlates and conundrums within and across cultures. *Social Science & Medicine, 45*(8), 1161–1176.

Fisher, M. (2012, June 28). Here's a map of the countries that provide universal health care (America's still not on it). *The Atlantic*. Retrieved from http://www.theatlantic.com/international/archive/2012/0krafft6/heres-a-map-of-the-countries-that-provide-universal-health-care-americas-still-not-on-it/259153/.

Fitzpatrick, M. (2004). From 'nanny state' to 'therapeutic state.' *The British Journal of General Practice, 54*(505), 645.

Flynn, T. (2006). The ties that [don't] bind: Transgender family law and the unmaking of Families. In P. Currah, R. M. Juang & S. P. Minter (Eds.), *Transgender rights* (pp. 32–50). Minneapolis: University of Minnesota Press.

Foster, E. (2008). Commitment, communication, and contending with heteronormativity: An invitation to greater reflexivity in interpersonal research. *Southern Communication* Journal, *73*(1), 84–101.

Foucault, M. (1990). *The history of sexuality: An introduction*. New York, NY: Vintage Books.

Fouratt, J. (2003, May 23–29). Thousands mourn Sakia: Lesbian teens rally around a sister lost to a hate crime. *Gay City News*. Retrieved from http://web.archive.org/web/20041215233118/http://www.gaycitynews.com/gcn221/thousandsmorn.html.

Franke, R., & Leary, M. R. (1991). Disclosure of sexual orientation by lesbian and gay men: A comparison of private and public processes. *Journal of Social and Clinical Psychology, 10*(3), 262–269.

Frankowski, B. (2004). Sexual orientation and adolescents. *Pediatrics, 113*(6), 1827–1832.

Freedom to Marry. (2013). States. Retrieved from http://www.freedomtomarry.org/states.

Frost, D. M. (2011). Stigma and intimacy in same-sex relationships: A narrative approach. *Journal of Family Psychology, 25*(1), 1–10.

Fugate, M., Landis, L., Riordan, K., Naureckas, S., & Engel, B. (2005). Barriers to domestic violence help seeking implications for intervention. *Violence Against Women, 11*(3), 290–310.

Gandhi, S., Rovi, S., Vega, M., Johnson, M. S., Ferrante, J., & Chen, P. H. (2010). Intimate partner violence and cancer screening among urban minority women. *Journal of the American Board of Family Medicine, 23*(3), 343–353.

Gates, G. J. (2011). *How many people are lesbian, gay, bisexual and transgender?* Special report by The Williams Institute. Retrieved from http://williamsinstitute.law.ucla.edu/wp-content/uploads/Gates-How-Many-People-LGBT-Apr-2011.pdf.

Gates, G., & Steinberger, M. D. (2009, May). *Same-sex unmarried partner couples in the American Community Survey: The role of misreporting, miscoding and misallocation*. Paper presented at the Annual Meeting of the Population Association of America, Detroit, MI. Retrieved from http://economics-files.pomona.edu/steinberger/research/Gates_Steinberger_ACS_Miscode_May2010.pdf.

Gay, Lesbian, and Straight Education Network. (2002). *The Day of Silence 2003 organizing manual.* Retrieved from http://web.archive.org/web/20030308002106/http://www.dayofsilence.org/downloads/organizingmanual.pdf.

Gay, Lesbian, and Straight Education Network. (2003). *April 9, 2003 Day of Silence.* Retrieved from http://www.dayofsilence.org/content/ra.html.

Gay, Lesbian, and Straight Education Network. (2007). *Resource usage agreement.* Retrieved from http://www.dayofsilence.org/content/ra.html.

Gay, Lesbian, and Straight Education Network. (2011a). *The Day of Silence organizing manual.* Retrieved from http://web.archive.org/web/20130518014535/http://dayofsilence.org/downloads/2011_DOS_Manual_FINAL.pdf.

Gay, Lesbian, and Straight Education Network. (2011b). *The history of the Day of Silence.* Retrieved from http://www.dayofsilence.org/content/history.html.

Gehi, P. S. (2009). Struggles from the margins: Anti-immigrant legislation and the impact on low-income transgender people of color. *Women's Rights Law Reporter 30,* 315–346.

Gehi, P. S., & Arkles, G. (2007). Unraveling injustice: Race and class impact of Medicaid exclusions of transition-related health care for transgender people. *Sexuality Research & Social Policy, 4*(4), 7–35.

Ginsburg, F., & Rapp, R. (1995). *Conceiving the new world order: The global politics of reproduction.* Berkeley, CA: University of California Press.

Glesne, C. (1999). *Becoming qualitative researchers: An introduction* (2nd ed.). New York: Longman.

Goldberg, N. G., & Meyer, I. H. (2013). Sexual orientation disparities in history of intimate partner violence results from the California Health Interview Survey. *Journal of Interpersonal Violence, 28*(5), 1109–1118.

Goldkuhl, G., & Cronholm, S. (2003, March). *Multi-grounded theory—Adding theoretical grounding to grounded theory.* Paper presented at the 2nd European Conference on Research Methodology for Business and Management Studies (ECRM 2003). Reading, UK: Reading University.

Gonzales, F., & Espin, O. M. (1996). Latino men, Latina women and homosexuality. In R. P. Cabaj, & T. S. Stein (Eds.), *Textbook of Homosexuality and Mental Health* (pp. 583–602). Washington, DC: American Psychiatric.

Gonzales, G., & Blewett, L. A. National and state-specific health insurance disparities for adults in same-sex relationships. *American Journal of Public Health* (forthcoming).

Gonzalez, J. M., Alegría, M., Prihoda, T. J., Copeland, L. A., & Zeber, J. E. (2011). How the relationship of attitudes toward mental health treatment and service use differs by age, gender, ethnicity/race and education. *Social Psychiatry and Psychiatric Epidemiology, 46*(1), 45–57.

Goodenow, C., Szalacha, L., & Westheimer, K. (2006). School support groups, other school factors, and the safety of sexual minority students. *Psychology in the Schools, 43*(5), 573–589.

Gould, E. (2012). Employer-sponsored health insurance erosion accelerates in the recession. *International Journal of Health Services, 42*(3), 499–537.

Grace, S., & Britain, G. (1995). *Policing domestic violence in the 1990s.* Home Office Research Study. Great Britain: Home Office.

Grant, J. M., Mottet, L. A., & Tanis, J., Harrison, J., Herman, J. L., & Keisling, M. (2011). *Injustice at every turn: A report of the National Transgender Discrimination Survey.* Retrieved from http://www.thetaskforce.org/downloads/reports/reports/ntds_full.pdf.

Grant, J. M., Mottet, L. A., Tanis, J., Herman, J. L., Harrison, J., & Keisling, M. (2010). *National Transgender Discrimination Survey Report on health and health care.* Washington, DC: National Center for Transgender Equality and National Gay and Lesbian Task Force. Retrieved from http://transequality.org/PDFs/NTDSReportonHealth final.pdf.

Greene, B. (1994). Lesbian women of color: Triple jeopardy. In L. Comas-Diaz, & B. Greene (Eds.), *Women of color: Integrating ethnic and gender identities in psychotherapy* (pp. 389–427). New York: Guilford.

Greenwood, G. L., Relf, M. V., Huang, B., Pollack, L. M., Canchola, J. A., & Catania, J. A. (2002). Battering victimization among a probability-based sample of men who have sex with men. *American Journal of Public Health, 92*(12), 1964–1969.

Griffith, K. H., & Hebl, M. R. (2002). The disclosure dilemma for gay men and lesbians: "Coming out" at work. *Journal of Applied Psychology, 87*(6), 1191–1999.

Haas, A. P., Eliason, M., Mays, V. M., Mathy, R. M., Cochran, S. D., D'Augelli, A. R., et al. (2010). Suicide and suicide risk in lesbian, gay, bisexual, and transgender populations: Review and recommendations. *Journal of Homosexuality, 58*(1), 10–51.

Halady, S. W. (2013). Attempted suicide, LGBT identity, and heightened scrutiny. *The American Journal of Bioethics, 13*(3), 20–22.

Hale, C. J. (1997). Leatherdyke boys and their daddies: How to have sex without women or men. *Social Text, 52/53*(153/154), 223–236.

Hammersley, M. (2008). *Questioning qualitative inquiry: Critical essays.* Thousand Oaks, CA: Sage.

Harris Interactive Poll. *New National Survey shows top causes for delay by lesbians in obtaining health care.* Rochester, NY: Harris, March 11, 2005. Retrieved from http://www.mautnerproject.org/programs_and_services/research/305.cfm.

Harwood, J., & Sparks, L. (2003). Social identity and health: An intergroup communication approach to cancer. *Health Communication, 15*(2), 145–159.

Hatzenbuehler, M. L. (2009). How does sexual minority stigma "Get under the skin"? A psychological meditation framework. *Psychological Bulletin 135*(5), 707–730.

Hawker, D. S., & Boulton, M. J., (2000). Twenty years' research on peer victimization and psychosocial maladjustment: A meta-analytic review of cross-sectional studies. *Journal of Child Psychology and Psychiatry, 41*(4): 441–455.

Hearn, J. (1996). *Men's violence to known women: historical, everyday and theoretical constructions.* In Fawcett et al. (Eds.), *Violence and gender relations: Theories and interventions* (pp. 22–37). London, UK: Sage Publishers.

Hearn, J. (1998). *The violences of men: How men talk about and how agencies respond to men's violence to women:* London, UK: Sage Publishers.

Heath, R. A. (2006). *The Praeger handbook of transsexuality: Changing gender to match mindset.* Westport, CT: Praeger Publishers.

Heck, J. E., Sell, R. L., & Gorrin, S. S. (2006). Health care access among individuals involved in same-sex relationships. *American Journal of Public Health, 96*(6), 1111–1118.

Heise, L. (1994). Gender-based abuse: the global epidemic. *Cadernos de Sade Publica, 10 (Supplement 1)*, S135–S145.

Herbst, J. H., Jacobs, E. D., Finlayson, T. J., McKleroy, V. S., Neumann, M. S., & Crepaz, N. (2008). Estimating HIV prevalence and risk behaviors of transgender persons in the United States: A systematic review. *AIDS Behavior, 12,* 1–17.

Herek, G. M. (1990). The context of anti-gay violence: Notes on cultural and psychological heterosexism. *Journal of Interpersonal Violence, 5*(1), 316–333.

Heyman, J., Guillermina Nunez, G., & Talavera, V. (2009). Health care access and barriers for unauthorized immigrants in El Paso County, Texas. *Family and Community Health, 32*(1), 4–21.

Hire, R. O. (2007). An interview with Frank Rundle, M.D., In *American psychiatry and homosexuality: An oral history*, ed. Drescher, J. & Merlino, J.P. New York: Harrington Press.

Hitchcock, J. M., & Wilson, H. S. (1992). Personal risking: Lesbian self-disclosure of sexual orientation to professional health care providers. *Nursing Research, 41*(3), 178–183.

Holahan, J. (2010). The 2007–09 recession and health insurance coverage. *Health Affairs, 30*(1), 145–152.

Holahan, J., & Cook, A. (2008). The US economy and changes in health insurance coverage, 2000–2006. *Health Affairs, 27*(2), w135–w144.

Hollingsworth v. Perry, 000 U.S. 12–144 (2013).

Hooker, E. (1957). The adjustment of the male overt homosexual. *Journal of Projective Techniques, 21,* 18–31.

Hopson, M. C. (2011). *Notes from the talking drum: Exploring black communication and critical memory through intercultural communication contexts.* Cresskill, NJ: Hampton Press Inc.

Houry, D., Kaslow, N. J., & Thompson, M. P. (2005). Depressive symptoms in women experiencing intimate partner violence. *Journal of Interpersonal Violence, 20*(11), 1467–1477.

Huang, H. Y., Yang, W., & Omaye, S. T. (2011). Intimate partner violence, depression and overweight/obesity. *Aggression and Violent Behavior, 16*(2), 108–114.

Human Rights Campaign. (2002). *Corporate equality index 2002.* Retrieved from http://www.hrc.org/files/assets/resources/CorporateEqualityIndex_2002.pdf.

Human Rights Campaign. (2011). *Growing up LGBT in America.* Retrieved from http://www.hrc.org/resources.

Human Rights Campaign. (2013a). *Growing up LGBT in America.* Retrieved from http://www.hrc.org/youth/about-the-survey-report#.UmsVOCQmymk.

Human Rights Campaign. (2013b). *Marriage equality and other relationship recognition laws.* Retrieved from http://www.hrc.org/files/assets/resources/marriage_equality_laws_072013.pdf.

Human Rights Campaign. (2013c). *An overview of federal rights and protections granted to married couples.* Retrieved from http://www.hrc.org/resources/entry/an-overview-of-federal-rights-and-protections-granted-to-married-couples.

Human Rights Campaign. (2013d). *Corporate equality index 2013: Rating American workplaces on lesbian, gay, bisexual and transgender equality.* Retrieved from http://www.hrc.org/corporate-equality-index/.

Hyde, H. M. (1970). *The love that dared not speak its name: A candid history of homosexuality in Britain.* Boston: Little Brown.

Ida, D. (2007). Cultural competency and recovery within diverse populations. *Psychiatric Rehabilitation Journal, 31*(1), 49–53.

Institute of Medicine. (2011). *The health of lesbian, gay, bisexual, and transgender people: Building a foundation for better understanding.* Washington, DC: National Academies Press.

Jackson, R. L. (2002). Cultural contracts theory: Toward an understanding of identity negotiation. *Communication Quarterly, 50*(3), 359–367.

Jeffries, S., & Ball, M. (2008). Male same-sex intimate partner violence: A descriptive review and call for further research. *Murdoch eLaw Review, 15*(1), 134–179.

Johnson, B. R., Oxendine, S., Taub, D. J., & Robertson, J. (2013). Suicide prevention for LGBT students. *New Directions for Student Services, 141*(March), 55–69.

Johnson, M. O., Carrico, A. W., Chesney, M. A., & Morin, S. F. (2008). Internalized heterosexism among HIV-positive, gay-identified men: Implications for HIV prevention and care. *Journal of Consulting and Clinical Psychology, 76*(5), 829–839.

Johnson, M., Smyer, T., & Yucha, C. (2012). Methodological quality of quantitative lesbian, gay, bisexual, and transgender nursing research from 2000 to 2010. *Advances in Nursing Science, 35*(2), 154–165.

Johnson, S. R., Guenther, S. M., Laube, D. W., & Keettel, W. C. (1981). Factors influencing lesbian gynecologic care: A preliminary study. *American Journal of Obstetrics and Gynecology, 140*(1), 20–28.

Jones, E. (1957). *Sigmund Freud: Life and work, Vol. 3: The last phase 1919–1939.* London: Hogarth Press.

Jones, L., Hughes, M., & Unterstaller, U. (2001). Post-Traumatic Stress Disorder (PTSD) in victims of domestic violence: A review of the research. *Trauma, Violence, & Abuse, 2*(2), 99–119.

Jüttner, J. (2013). *Gericht zu künstlicher Befruchtung: Vater wider Willen.* Retrieved from http://www.spiegel.de/panorama/justiz/kuenstliche-befruchtung-olg-hamm-weist-klage-eines-vaters-ab-a-881353.html.

Kanavos, P., & Gemmill-Toyama, M. (2010). Prescription drug coverage among elderly and disabled Americans: Can Medicare–Part D reduce inequities in access? *International Journal of Health Care Finance and Economics, 10*(3), 202–218.

Kanuha, V. K. (2000). 'Being' native versus 'going native': Conducting social work research as an insider. *Social Work, 45*(5): 439–447.

Kaufman, J. M., & Johnson, C. (2004). Stigmatized individuals and the process of identity. *The Sociological Quarterly, 45*(4), 807–833.

Kaufman, M. (1987). *The construction of masculinity and the triad of men's violence.* In Michael Kaufman (Ed.), *Beyond patriarchy: Essays by men on pleasure, power, and change* (pp. 1–29). Toronto, Canada: Oxford University Press.

Kay, M., & Jeffries, S. (2010). Homophobia, heteronormativism and hegemonic masculinity: Male same-sex intimate violence from the perspective of Brisbane service providers. *Psychiatry, Psychology and Law, 17*(3), 412–423.

Keller, S. E. (1999). Crisis of authority: Medical rhetoric and transsexual identity. *Yale Journal of Law and Feminism, 11*(51), 51–74.

Kelley, T. (2003, May 14). New Jersey: Newark: Warrant issued for arrest in stabbing. *The New York Times*, p. 5.

Kelly, R. C. (2012). *Borders that matter: Trans identity management*. (Unpublished doctoral dissertation). University at Albany, State University of New York, Albany, NY.

Kenagy, G. R. (2005). Transgender health: Findings from two needs assessment studies in Philadelphia. *Health & Social Work, 30*(1), 19–26.

Keyton, J. (2005). *Communication research: Asking questions, finding answers*. New York, NY: McGraw-Hill.

Kidd, J., & Witten, T. (2008). Transgender and transsexual identities: The next strange fruit—Hate crimes, violence and genocide against the global trans-communities. *Journal of Hate Studies, 6*(31), 31–63.

Killermann, S. (2013). *The social justice advocate's handbook: A guide to gender*. Retrieved from http://www.guidetogender.com/.

Kim, H.-J., & Fredriksen-Goldsen, K. I. (2012). Hispanic lesbians and bisexual women at heightened risk of health disparities. *American Journal of Public Health, 102(1)*, 9–15. doi: 10.2105/AJPH.2011.300378.

King, E. B., Reilly, C., & Hebl, M. (2008). The best of times, the worst of times: Exploring dual perspectives of 'coming out' in the workplace. *Group and Organization Management, 33*(5), 566–601.

Kinsey, A., Pomeroy, W. B. & Martin, C. E. (1948). *Sexual behavior in the human male*. Philadelphia: W. B. Saunders.

Kinsey, A., Pomeroy, W., Martin, C., and Gebhard, P. (1953). *Sexual behavior in the human female*. Philadelphia: W. B. Saunders.

Kitzinger, C. (2009). Doing gender: A conversation analytic perspective. *Gender & Society, 23*(1), 94–98.

Klein, E. (2012, June 24). 11 facts about the Affordable Care Act. *The Washington Post*. Retrieved from http://www.washingtonpost.com/blogs/wonkblog/wp/2012/06/24/11–facts-about-the-affordable-care-act/.

Klostermann, K., Kelley, M. L., Milletich, R. J., & Mignone, T. (2011). Alcoholism and partner aggression among gay and lesbian couples. *Aggression and Violent Behavior, 16*(2),115–119.

Kosciw, J. G., Greytak, E. A., Bartkiewicz, M. J., Boesen, M. J., & Palmer, N. A. (2012). *The 2011 National School Climate Survey: The experiences of lesbian, gay, bisexual, and transgender youth in our nation's schools*. New York: GLSEN.

Kosciw, J. G., Palmer, N. A., Kull, R. M., & Greytak, E. A. (2013). The effect of negative school climate on academic outcomes for LGBT youth and the role of in-school supports. *Journal of School Violence, 12*(1), 45–63.

Kovach, K. (2004). Trauma nursing: Intimate partner violence. *RN, 67*(8), 38–43.

Koziol-McLain, J., Gardiner, J., Batty, P., Rameka, M., Fyfe, E., & Giddings, L. (2004). Prevalence of intimate partner violence among women presenting to an urban adult and paediatric emergency care department. *New Zealand Medical Journal: Journal Of The New Zealand Medical Association, 117*(1206), U1174.

Krafft-Ebbing, von R. (1886). *Psychopathia Sexualis—Contrary sexual instinct: A medico-legal study*. London: R.J. Rebman.

Krehely, J. (2009, December 1). How to close the LGBT health disparities gap. *Center for American Progress.* Retrieved from http://www.americanprogress.org/issues/lgbt/report/2009/12/21/7048/how-to-close-the-lgbt-health-disparities-gap/.

Kronemeyer, R. (1980). *Overcoming homosexuality.* New York: Macmillan.

Kus, R. J. (1985). Stages of coming out: An ethnographic approach. *Western Journal of Nursing Research, 7*(2), 177–198.

Lambda Legal. (2013a). *Adoption and parenting.* Retrieved from http://www.lambdalegal.org/issues/adoption-and-parenting

Lambda Legal. (2013b). *Status of same-sex relationships nationwide.* Retrieved from http://www.lambdalegal.org/publications/nationwide-status-same-sex-relationships#2.

Lehavot, K., Walters, K. L., & Simoni, J. M. (2010). Abuse, mastery, and health among lesbian, bisexual, and two-spirit American Indian and Alaska Native women. *Cultural Diversity and Ethnic Minority Psychology, 15*(3), 275–284.

Lehman, M. (1997). At the end of the rainbow: A report on gay male domestic violence and abuse. *Minnesota Center Against Violence and Abuse,* http://www.mincava.umn.edu/documents/rainbow/At The End Of The Rainbow.pdf.

Lehmann, J. B., Lehmann, C. U., & Kelly, P. J. (1998). Development and health care needs of lesbians. *Journal of Women's Health, 7*(3), 379–387.

Lewes, K. (2009). *Psychoanalysis and male homosexuality: Twentieth-anniversary edition.* Plymouth: Jason Aronson.

Lewis, R. J., Derlega, V. J., Griffin, J. L., & Krowinski, A. C. (2003). Stressors for gay men and lesbians: Life stress, gay-related stress, stigma consciousness, and depressive symptoms. *Journal of Social and Clinical Psychology, 22*(6), 716–729.

Lindlof, T. R., & Taylor, B. C. (2002). *Qualitative communication research methods.* Thousand Oaks, CA: Sage.

Lindlof, T. R., & Taylor, B. C. (2011). *Qualitative communication research methods (3rd ed).* Thousand Oaks, CA: Sage.

Liu, R. T., & Mustanski, B. (2012). Suicidal ideation and self-harm in lesbian, gay, bisexual, and transgender youth. *American Journal of Preventive Medicine, 42*(3), 221–228.

Lloyd, B., Ennis, F., & Alkinson, T. (1994). *The power of women-positive literacy work: Program-based action research.* Halifax, NS: Fernwood.

Logie, C., Bridge, T. J., & Bridge, P. D. (2007). Evaluating the phobias, attitudes, and cultural competence of master of social work students toward the LGBT populations. *Journal of Homosexuality, 53*(4), 201–221.

Loiacano, D. (1989). Gay identity issues among Black Americans: Racism, homophobia, and the need for validation. *Journal of Counseling & Development, 68*(1), 21–25.

Lorde, A. (1984). The transformation of silence into language and action. In A. Lorde (Ed.), *Sister outsider: Essays and speeches* (pp. 40–44). Trumansburg, NY: Crossing Press.

Lucal, B. (1999). What it means to be gendered me: Life on the boundaries of a dichotomous gender system. *Gender & Society, 13*(6), 781–797.

Lunceford, B. (2011). Must we all be rhetorical historians? Relevance and timliness in rhetorical scholarship. *Journal of Contemporary Rhetoric, 1*(1), 1–9.

Manning, J. (In press). Communicating sexual identities: A typology of coming out conversations. *Communication Quarterly*.

Manning, J. (2006). *Exploring coming out narratives: Toward a communicative theory of the coming out process* (Doctoral dissertation). Retrieved from *ProQuest Dissertations and Theses* (Order No. 3222189).

Manning, J. (2009). Because the personal is the political: Politics and unpacking the rhetoric of (queer) relationships. In B. Drushel, & K. German (Eds.), *Queer identities/ political realities* (pp. 1–8). Newcastle, UK: Cambridge Scholars.

Manning, J. (2009). Heterosexuality. In J. O'Brien (Ed.), *Encyclopedia of gender and society* (pp. 413–417). Thousand Oaks, CA: Sage.

Manning, J. (2010). 'There is no agony like bearing an untold story inside you': Communication research as interventive practice. *Communication Monographs, 77*(4), 437–439. doi:10.1080/03637751.2010.523596.

Manning, J. (2011). Sexual orientation. In M. Z. Stange, C. K. Oyster, & J. G. Golson (Eds.), *The encyclopedia of women in today's world* (pp. 1319–1321). Thousand Oaks, CA: Sage.

Manning, J. (2013). Interpretive theorizing in the seductive world of sexuality and interpersonal communication: Getting guerilla with studies of sexting and purity rings. *International Journal of Communication, 7*.

Manning, J. (2014). Communication and healthy sexual practices: Toward a holistic communicology of sexuality. In M. H. Eaves (Ed.), *Applications in health communication: Emerging trends*. Dubuque, IA: Kendall-Hunt.

Manning, J. (2014). A constitutive approach to interpersonal communication studies. *Communication Studies, 65*(3).

Manning, J. (2014). Perceptions of positive and negative communicative behaviors in coming out conversations. *Journal of Homosexuality*.

Manning, J. (2014). Values in online and offline dating discourses: Comparing presentational and articulated rhetorics of relationship seeking. *Journal of Computer-Mediated Communication, 19*(2).

Manning, J., & Kunkel, A. (2014). *Researching interpersonal relationships: Qualitative methods, studies, and analysis*. Thousand Oaks, CA: Sage Publications.

Manning, J., Vlasis, M., Dirr, J., Shandy, A., Emerson, T., & De Paz, T. (2008). (Inter)(cross)(multi)(trans)disciplining sex, gender, and sexuality studies: A qualitative inquiry into the reflections of researchers, teachers, and practitioners. *Women & Language, 31*(2), 36–41.

Marrazzo, J. M., Coffey, P., & Bingham, A. (2005). Sexual practices, risk perception and knowledge of sexually transmitted disease risk among lesbian and bisexual women. *Perspectives on Sexual and Reproductive Health, 37*(1), 6–12.

Marrazzo, J. M., & Gorgos, L. M. (2012). Emerging sexual health issues among women who have sex with women. *Current Infectious Disease Reports, 14*, 204–211.

Marshall, M., Friedman, M. S., Stall, R. and Thompson, A. L. (2009). Individual trajectories of substance use in lesbian, gay and bisexual youth and heterosexual youth. *Addiction, 104*(6), 974–981.

Max, W., Rice, D. P., Finkelstein, E., Bardwell, R. A., & Leadbetter, S. (2004). The economic toll of intimate partner violence against women in the United States. *Violence and Victims, 19*(3), 259–272.

Maxwell, J. A. (2013). *Qualitative research design: An interactive approach.* Thousand Oaks, CA: Sage.

May, E. T. (1988). *Homeward bound: American families in the Cold War Era.* New York: Basic Books.

Maykut, P., & Morehouse, R. (1994). *Beginning qualitative researchers: A philosophical and practical guide.* Washington, DC: Falmer.

Mays, V. M., & Cochran, S. D. (2001). Mental health correlates of perceived discrimination among lesbian, gay, and bisexual adults in the United States. *American Journal of Public Health, 91*(11), 1869–76.

McCauley, J., Kern, D. E., Kolodner, K., Dill, L., Schroeder, A. F., DeChant, H. K., et al. (1995). The 'battering syndrome': Prevalence and clinical characteristics of domestic violence in primary care internal medicine practices. *Annals of Internal Medicine, 123*(10), 737–746.

McClennen, J. C. (2005). Domestic violence between same-gender partners recent findings and future research. *Journal of Interpersonal Violence, 20*(2), 149–154.

McClennen, J. C., Summers, A. B., & Vaughan, C. (2002). Gay men's domestic violence: Dynamics, help-seeking behaviors, and correlates. *Journal of Gay & Lesbian Social Services, 14*(1), 23–49.

McCormick, B. (1994). Anti-gay discrimination impedes careers, health care. *American Medical News, 37*(26), 7.

McFarlane, J., Malecha, A., Watson, K., Gist, J., Batten, E., Hall, I., et al. (2005). Intimate partner sexual assault against women: Frequency, health consequences, and treatment outcomes. *Obstetrics & Gynecology, 105*(1), 99–108.

McGrath, J. J. (2004). Abstinence-only adolescent education: Ineffective, unpopular and unconstitutional. *Bepress Legal Series, 150.*

Meenan, M. (2003a, November 27–December 3). Rare bias indictment in Sakia Gunn murder. *Gay City News.* Retrieved from http://gaycitynews.com/gcn_248/rarebias .html.

Meenan, M. (2003b, May 23–29). Tears and then, perhaps, respect: As thousands of Newark's youth mourn, the city scrambles to respond. *Gay City News.* Retrieved from http://web.archive.org/web/20051024122904/http://www.gaycitynews.com/gcn221/tearsandthen.html.

Meenan, M. (2005, March 10–16). Sakia Gunn's killer pleads guilty. *Gay City News.* Retrieved from http://gaycitynews.com/gcn_410/sakiagunnskiller.html.

Mercer. (2012). *Employers held health benefit cost growth to 4.1% in 2012, the smallest increase in 15 years.* Retrieved from http://www.mercer.com/press-releases/1491670.

Merrill, G. S., & Wolfe, V. A. (2000). Battered gay men: An exploration of abuse, help seeking, and why they stay. *Journal of Homosexuality, 39*(2), 1–30.

Messinger, A. M. (2011). Invisible victims: Same-sex IPV in the national violence against women survey. *Journal of Interpersonal Violence, 26*(11), 2228–2243.

Messner, M. A., & Sabo, D. F. (1994). *Sex, violence & power in sports: Rethinking masculinity.* Freedom, CA: The Crossing Press.

Meyer, I. H. (1995). Minority stress and mental health in gay men. *Journal of Health and Social Behavior, 36*(1), 38–56.

Meyer, I. H. (2003). Prejudice, social stress, and mental health in lesbian, gay, and bisexual populations: Conceptual issues and research evidence. *Psychological Bulletin, 129*(5). 674–697.

Meyerowtiz, J. (2002). *How sex changed: A history of transsexuality in the United States.* Cambridge, MA: Harvard University Press.

Milar, K. S. (2011). The myth buster: Evelyn Hooker's groundbreaking research exploded the notion that homosexuality was a mental illness, ultimately removing it from the DSM. *Monitor on Psychology, 42*(2), 24.

Minnesota Population Center and State Health Access Data Assistance Center. (2012). *Integrated health interview series: Version 5.0.* Minneapolis: University of Minnesota. Retrieved from http://ihis.us.

Minton, H. L. (2002). *Departing from deviance: A history of homosexual rights and emancipatory science in America.* Chicago: University of Chicago Press.

Mogul, J. L., Ritchie, A. J., & Whitlock, K. (2011). *Queer (in)hjustice.* Boston, MA: Beacon Press.

Mohr, J. J., & Daly, C. A. (2008). Sexual minority stress and changes in relationship quality in same-sex couples. *Journal of Social and Personal Relationships, 25*(6), 989–1007.

Movement Advancement Project's "2009 Momentum Report" (2009). Retrieved from https://www.lgbtmap.org/ momentum-report.html.

Moyer, C. S. (2011, September 5). LGBT patients: reluctant and underserved. *American Medical News.* Retrieved from http://www.amednews.com/article/20110905/profession/309059942/4/.

Moyer, V. A. (2013). Screening for HIV: U.S. Preventative Services Task Force recommendation statement. *Annals of Internal Medicine, 159*(1), 51–60.

msn.com. (2013). Where gay marriage stands in all 50 states. Retrieved from http://news.msn.com/us/where-gay-marriage-stands-in-all-50–states.

Mucciaroni, G. (2008). *Same sex, different politics: Success and failure in the struggles over gay rights.* University Chicago Press, London.

Mueller, T. E., Gavin, L. E., & Kulkarni, A. (2008). The association between sex education and youth's engagement in sexual intercourse, age at first intercourse, and birth control use at first sex. *Journal of Adolescent Health, 42*(1), 89–96.

Mulligan, E., & Heath, M. (2007). Seeking open minded doctors: How women who identify as bisexual, queer or lesbian seek quality health care. *Australian Family Physician, 36*(6), 469–471.

Mullings, B. (1999). Insider or outsider, both or neither: Some dilemmas of interviewing in a cross-cultural setting. *Geoforum, 30*(4), 337–350.

Mustanski, B. S. (2001). Getting wired: Exploiting the Internet for the collection of valid sexuality data. *Journal of Sex Research 38*(4), 292–301.

Mustanski, B. S., Garofalo, R., & Emerson, E. M. (2010). Mental health disorders, psychological distress, and suicidality in a diverse sample of lesbian, gay, bisexual, and transgender youths. *American Journal of Public Health, 100*(12), 2426–2432.

Mustanski, B., & Liu, R. T., (2013). A longitudinal study of predictors of suicide attempts among lesbian, gay, bisexual, and transgender youth. *Archives of Sexual Behavior, 42*(3), 437–448.

Nadal, K. L., Skolnik, A., & Wong, Y. (2012). Interpersonal and systemic microaggressions toward transgender people: Iemplications for counseling. *Journal of LBGT Issues in Counseling, 6*(1), 55–82.

Namaste, V. (2000). *Invisible lives: The erasure of transsexual and transgender people.* Chicago: University of Chicago Press.

National Center for Health Statistics. (2012a). *Health, United States* (Library of Congress Catalog No 76–641496). Hyattsville, MD: National Center for Health Statistics. Retrieved from http://www.cdc.gov/nchs/data/hus/hus12.pdf.

National Center for Health Statistics. (2012b). *Multiple imputation of family income and personal earnings in the national health interview survey: Methods and examples.* Retrieved from http://www.cdc.gov/nchs/data/nhis/tecdoc11.pdf.

National Coalition for LGBT Health. (2010). *Report on the United States of America: Universal Periodic Review of Sexual Rights, 9th Round.* Washington, DC: The National Coalition of LGBT Health.

National Patient Safety Foundation. (2013). *Ask me 3.* Retrieved from http://www.npsf.org/for-healthcare-professionals/programs/ask-me-3/.

National Survey of Substance Abuse Treatment Services (2010, June). *Substance abuse treatment programs for gays and lesbians.* Retrieved from http://www.samhsa.gov/data/spotlight/Spotlight004GayLesbians.pdf.

NBC. (2010, September 9). Number of uninsured Americans hits record high. *NBC. com.* Retrieved from http://www.nbcnews.com/id/39215770/ns/health-health_care/t/number-uninsured-americans-hits-record-high/#.UkSQ9LyhtNI.

Nemoto, T., Bodeker, B., & Iwamoto, M. (2011). Social support, exposure to violence, and transphobia: Correlates of depression among male-to-female transgender women with a history of sex work. *American Journal of Public Health, 101,* 1980–1988.

Newfield, E., Hart, S., Dibble, S., & Kohler, L. (2006). Female-to-male transgender quality of life. *Quality of Life Research, 15,* 1447–1457.

NOLO Law for All. (2013). Law prohibiting discrimination against gays and lesbians FAQ. *NOLO Law for All.* Retrieved from http://www.nolo.com/legal-encyclopedia/laws-prohibiting-discrimination-against-gays-faq-32295.html.

Nordmarken, S. (2013, March). *Disrupting gendering: How trans and gender variant people interrupt and transfigure the gender accomplishment process.* Paper presented at the annual meeting of the Eastern Sociological Society. Boston, MA.

O'Connell, M., & Feliz, S. (2011). *Same-sex couples household statistics from the 2010 Census* (Social, Economic and Housing Statistics Working Paper 2011–26).Washington, DC: U.S. Bureau of the Census.

O'Connell, M., & Gooding, G. (2007). *Editing unmarried couples in Census Bureau data* (Housing and Household Economic Statistics Division Working Paper). Washington, DC: U.S. Bureau of the Census. Retrieved from http://www.census.gov/population/www/documentation/twps07/twps07.html.

O'Hanlan, K. A., Dibble S. L., Hagan, J. J., & Davids, R. (2004). Advocacy for women's health should include lesbian health. *Journal of Women's Health, 13*(2), 227–234.

Orr, D. P., Beiter, M., Ingersoll, G. M. (1991). Premature sexual activity is an indicator of psychosocial risk. *Pediatrics, 87*(2), 141–147.

Otis, M. D., Rostosky, S. S., Riggle, E. D., & Hamrin, R. (2006). Stress and relationship quality in same-sex couples. *Journal of Social and Personal Relationships, 23*(1), 81–99.

Owen, W. (1984). Interpretative themes in relational communication. *Quarterly Journal of Speech, 70,* 274–287.

Parker-Pope, T. (2009, May 19). Kept from a dying partner's bedside. *The New York Times,* p. D5.

Patton, M. Q. (2002). *Qualitative research & evaluation methods.* Thousand Oaks, CA: Sage.

Pauly, I. B. (1990). Gender identity disorders: Evaluation and treatment. *Journal of Sex Education and Therapy, 16*(1), 2–24.

Pawson, R. (1996). Theorizing the interview. *The British Journal of Sociology 47*(2), 295–314.

Pearson, K. (2006). Small murders: Rethinking news coverage of hate crimes against GLBT people. In L. Castañeda & S. B. Campbell (Eds.), *News and sexuality: Media portraits of diversity* (pp. 159–190). Thousand Oaks, CA: Sage Publications.

Peckover, S. (2003). 'I could have just done with a little more help': An analysis of women's help seeking from health visitors in the context of domestic violence. *Health & Social Care in the Community, 11*(3), 275–282.

Peplau, L. A., & Garnets, L. D. (2000). A new paradigm for understanding women's sexuality and sexual orientation. *Journal of Social Issues, 56*(2), 330–350.

Petronio, S., & Sargent, J. (2011). Disclosure predicaments arising during the course of patient care: Nurses' privacy management. *Health Communication, 26*(3), 255–266. doi:10.1080/10410236.2010.549812.

Pilkington, N. W., & D'Augelli, A. R. (1995). Victimization of lesbian, gay and bisexual youth in community settings. *Journal of Community Psychology, 23*(1), 34–56.

Pizer, J. C., Sears, B., Mallory, C., & Hunter, N. D. (2012). Evidence of persistent and pervasive workplace discrimination against LGBT people: The need for federal legislation prohibiting discrimination and providing equal employment benefits. *Layola of Los Angeles Law Review. Loyola of Las Angeles Law Review, 45*(3), 715–780.

Plichta, S. B. (2004). Intimate partner violence and physical health consequences policy and practice implications. *Journal of Interpersonal Violence, 19*(11), 1296–1323.

Plichta, S. B. (2007). Interactions between victims of intimate partner violence against women and the health care system policy and practice implications. *Trauma, Violence, & Abuse, 8*(2), 226–239.

Plummer, K. (1995). *Telling sexual stories: Power, change, and social worlds.* New York: Routledge.

Polek, C., & Hardie, T. (2010). Lesbian women and knowledge about human papillomavirus. *Oncology Nursing Forum, 37*(3), E191–E197.

Poorman, P. B., Seelau, E. P., & Seelau, S. M. (2003). Perceptions of domestic abuse in same-sex relationships and implications for criminal justice and mental health responses. *Violence and Victims, 18*(6), 659–669.

Porcerelli, J. H., Cogan, R., West, P. P., Rose, E. A., Lambrecht, D., Wilson, K. E., et al. (2003). Violent victimization of women and men: Physical and psychiatric symptoms. *The Journal of the American Board of Family Practice, 16*(1), 32–39.

President's Council on Bioethics. (2011). *Reproduction and responsibility: The regulation of new biotechnologies.* Washington, DC: US Government Printing Office.

Rado, S. (1940). A critical examination of the concept of bisexuality. *Psychosomatic Medicine, 2,* 459–467.

Ramsay, J., Richardson, J., Carter, Y. H., Davidson, L. L., & Feder, G. (2002). Should health professionals screen women for domestic violence? Systematic review. *Bmj, 325*(7359), 314.

Ramsey, G. (1996). *Transsexuals: Candid answers to private questions.* Freedom, CA: Crossing Press.

Rankow, E. J. (1995). Lesbian health issues for the primary care provider. *Journal of Family Practice, 40*(5), 486–493.

Rauprich, O., Berns, E., & Vollmann, J. (2010). Who should pay for assisted reproductive techniques? Answers from patients, professionals and the general public in Germany. *Human Reproduction, 25*(5), 1225–1233. doi: 10.1093/humrep/deq056.

Remafedi, G. (Ed.). (1994). *Death by denial: Studies of suicide in gay and lesbian teenagers.* Boston: Alyson Publications.

Rennison, C. M., & Welchans, S. (2003). *Intimate partner violence.* Washington DC: Bureau of Justice.

Resolve. (2013). *Health insurance 101.* Retrieved from http://www.resolve.org/family-building-options/insurance_coverage/health-insurance-101.html.

Richardson, J., Coid, J., Petruckevitch, A., Chung, W. S., Moorey, S., & Feder, G. (2002). Identifying domestic violence: Cross sectional study in primary care. *Bmj, 324*(7332), 274.

Richardt, N. (2003). A comparative analysis of the embryological research debate in Great Britain and Germany. *Social Politics: International Studies in Gender, State and Society, 10*(1), 86–128. http://sp.oxfordjournals.org/.

Rienzo, B. A., Button, J. W. Sheu, J., & Li, Y. (2006). The politics of sexual orientation issues in American schools. *Journal of School Health, 76*(3), 93–97.

Rivers, I. (2004). Recollections of bullying at school and their long-term implications for lesbians, gay men, and bisexuals. *Crisis, 25*(4), 169–175.

Robertson, J. A. (2004). Reproductive technology in Germany and the United States: An essay in comparative law and bioethics. *Columbia Journal of Transnational Law 43,* 189–227.

Rosario, M., Schrimshaw, E. W., Hunter, J., & Braun, L. (2006). Sexual identity development among lesbian, gay, and bisexual youths: Consistency and change over time. *The Journal of Sex Research, 43*(1), 46–58.

Rose, P. (1985). *Writing on women: Essays in a renaissance.* Middletown, CT: Wesleyan University Press.

Roszak, T. (2009). *The making of an elder culture.* Gabriola Island, BC, Canada: New Society Publishers.

Roter, D., & Hall, J. A. (2006). *Doctors talking with patients/patients talking with doctors: Improving communication in medical visits* (2nd ed.). Westport, CT: Greenwood.

Russ, T. L., Simonds, C. J., & Hunt, S. K. (2002). Coming out in the classroom. . . . An occupational hazard? The influence of sexual orientation on teacher credibility and perceived student learning. *Communication Education, 51*(3), 311–324.

Russell, S. T., Ryan, C., Toomey, R. B., Diaz, R. M., & Sanchez, J. (2011). Lesbian, gay, bisexual, and transgender adolescent school victimization: Implications for young adult health and adjustment. *Journal of School Health, 81*(5), 223–230.

Rust, P. C. (1996). "Coming out" in the age of social constructionism: Sexual identity formation among lesbian and bisexual women. *Journal of Lesbian Studies, 1*(1), 25–54.

Rust, P. C. (2003). Finding a sexual identity and community: Therapeutic implications and cultural assumptions in scientific models of coming out. In L. D. Garnets, & D. C. Kimmel (Eds.), *Psychological perspectives on lesbian, gay and bisexual experiences* (pp. 227–69). New York: Columbia University Press.

Roth, K. A., Mefford, I. M., & Barchas, J. D. (1982). Epinephrine, norepinephrine, dopamine and serotonin: Differential effects of acute and chronic stress on regional brain amines. *Brain Research, 239*(2), 417–424.

Sanchez, N. F., Sanchez, J. P., & Danoff, A. (2009). Health care utilization, barriers to care, and hormone usage among male-to-female transgender persons in New York City. *American Journal of Public Health, 99*(4), 713–19.

Schilt, K., & Westbrook, L. (2009). "Gender normals," transgender people, and the social maintenance of heterosexuality. *Gender & Society, 23*(4), 440–464.

Schmid, S. (2009). Assisted reproduction in Switzerland and Germany: Regulative and social contexts. In W. De Jong & O. Tkach (Eds.), *Making bodies, persons and families: Normalising reproductive technologies in Russia, Switzerland and Germany* (57–72). Piscataway, NJ: Transaction Publishers.

Schope, R. D. (2002). The decision to tell: Factors influencing the disclosure of sexual orientation by gay men. *Journal of Gay & Lesbian Social Services, 14*(1), 1–22.

Schrock, D., Boyd, E. M., & Leaf, M. (2007). Emotion work in the public performances of male-to-female transsexuals. *Archives of Sexual Behavior 38*(5), 702–712.

Scott, J. W. (1992). Experience. In J. Butler & J. W. Scott (Eds.), *Feminists theorize the political* (pp. 22–40). New York, NY: Routledge.

Sedgwick, E. K. (1990). *Epistemology of the closet.* Berkeley, CA: University of California.

Serano, J. (2007). *Whipping girl: A transsexual woman on sexism and the scapegoating of femininity.* Emeryville, CA: Seal Press.

Shapiro, E. (2004). Trans'cending barriers: Transgender organizing on the Internet. *Journal of Gay and Lesbian Social Services 16,* 165–180.

Sheridan, V. (2009). *The complete guide to transgender in the workplace.* Santa Barbara, CA: ABC-CLIO, LLC.

Sherman, L. W., Smith, D. A., Schmidt, J. D., & Rogan, D. P. (1992). Crime, punishment, and stake in conformity: Legal and informal control of domestic violence. *American Sociological Review, 57*(5), 680–690.

Shernoff, M. (2005). The sociology of barebacking. *The Gay & Lesbian Review Worldwide, 7*(1), 33–35.

Shilo, G., & Savaya, R. (2011). Effects of family and friend support on LGB youths' mental health and sexual orientation milestones. *Family Relations, 60*(3), 318–330.

Silver, N. (2013, March 26). How opinion on same-sex marriage is changing, and what it means. *New York Times.* Retrieved from http://fivethirtyeight.blogs.

nytimes.com/2013/03/26/how-opinion-on-same-sex-marriage-is-changing-and-what-it-means/.

Silverman, D. (2013). *Doing qualitative research: A practical handbook.* London: Sage.

Skinner, C. J., Stokes, J., Kirlew Y., Kavanagh J., & Forster, G. E. (1996). A case-controlled study of the sexual health needs of lesbians. *Genitourinary Medicine, 72*(4), 277–280.

Sloop, J. M. (2000). Disciplining the transgendered: Brandon Teena, public representation, and normativity. *Western Journal of Communication, 64*(2), 165–189.

Smith, E. M., Johnson, S. R., & Guenther, S. M. (1985). Health care attitudes and experiences during gynecological care among lesbians and bisexuals. *American Journal of Public Health, 75*(9), 1085–1087.

Smith, D. M., Richman, D. D., & Little, S. J. (2005). HIV superinfection. *The Journal of Infectious Diseases, 192*(3), 438–444.

Smothers, R. (2003a, May 13). Teenage girl fatally stabbed at a bus stop in Newark. *The New York Times,* p. 8.

Smothers, R. (2003b, May 16). Man arrested in the killing of a teenager in Newark. *The New York Times,* p. 4.

Snyder, J. E. (2011). Trend analysis of medical publications about LGBT persons: 1950–2007. *Journal of Homosexuality, 58*(2), 164–188.

Snyder, J. E. (2011). Trend analysis of medical publications about LGBT persons: 1950–2007. *Journal of Homosexuality, 58*(2), 164–188.

Solarz, A. L. (Ed.). (1999). *Lesbian health: current assessment and directions for the future.* Washington, DC: National Academy Press.

Sourander, A, Jensen, P., Rönning, J. A., Niemelä, S., Helenius, H., Sillanmäki, L., Kumpulainen, K., Piha, J., Tamminen, T., Moilanen, I., & Almqvist, F. (2007). What is the early adulthood outcome of boys who bully or are bullied in childhood? The Finnish 'From a Boy to a Man' study. *Pediatrics, 120*(2), 397–404.

Southern Poverty Law Center. (2013). Hate incidents. Retrieved from http://www.splcenter.org/get-informed/hate-incidents.

Spade, D. (2011). *Normal life: Administrative violence, critical trans politics, and the limits of law.* New York: South End Press.

Speer, S. A., & Potter, J. (2000). The management of heterosexist talk: Conversationalist resources and prejudiced claims. *Discourse & Society, 11*(4), 543–572.

Spradley, J. P. (1979). *The ethnographic interview.* New York: Holt, Rinehart and Winston.

Spradlin, L. K. (2012). *Diversity matters: Understanding diversity in schools* (2nd ed.). Belmont, CA: Thomson/Wadsworth.

Sproul, K., LaVally, R., & Research, C. L. S. O. (1997). *California's response to domestic violence.* California Senate Office of Research.

Stanko, E. A. (1994). Challenging the problem of men's individual violence. In T. Newburn & E. A. Stanko (Eds.), *Just boys doing business?: Men, masculinities and crime* (pp. 32–450). London, England: Routledge.

State Health Access Data Assistance Center. (2013). *State-level trends in employer-sponsored insurance.* Minneapolis, MN: University of Minnesota. Retrieved from http://www.shadac.org/publications/state-level-trends-in-employer-sponsored-insurance.

St. Pierre, M. (2012). Under what conditions do lesbians disclose their sexual orientation to primary healthcare providers? A review of the literature. *Journal of Lesbian Studies, 16*(2), 199–219.

St. Pierre, M., & Senn, C. Y. (2010). External barriers to help-seeking encountered by Canadian gay and lesbian victims of intimate partner abuse: An application of the barriers model. *Violence and Victims, 25*(4), 536–552.

Stein, M. B., & Kennedy, C. (2001). Major depressive and post-traumatic stress disorder comorbidity in female victims of intimate partner violence. *Journal of Affective Disorders, 66*(2), 133–138.

Stevens, P. E. (1994). Lesbians' health-related experiences of care and noncare. *Western Journal of Nursing Research, 16*(6), 639–669.

Stevens, P. E. (1995). Structural and interpersonal impact of heterosexual assumptions on lesbian health care clients. *Nursing Research, 44*(1), 25–30.

Stevens, P. E., Tatum, N. O., & White, J. C. (1996). Optimal care for lesbian patients. *Patient Care*, March 15, 122–123.

Strauss, A., & Corbin, J. (1990). *Basics of qualitative research: Grounded theory procedures and techniques*. Thousand Oaks, CA: Sage.

Streitmatter, R. (2009). *From 'perverts' to 'fab five': The media's changing depiction of gay men and lesbians*. New York and London: Routledge Taylor & Francis Group.

Stryker, S. (2008). *Transgender history*. Emeryville, CA: Seal Press.

Sue, D. W. (2010). *Microaggressions and marginality: Manifestation, dynamics, and impact*. New Jersey: John Wiley & Sons.

Sun, L. H. (2013, September 25). Navigating the Affordable Care Act, whose health insurance exchanges open Tuesday. *The Washington Post*. Retrieved from http://www.washingtonpost.com/national/health-science/navigating-the-affordable-care-act-whose-health-insurance-exchanges-open-tuesday/2013/09/25/c1c7dcaa-2229-11e3-b73c-aab60bf735d0_story.html.

Surgenor, L. J. (1985). Attitudes toward seeking professional psychological help. *New Zealand Journal of Psychology, 14*: 27–33.

Swearer, S. M., Turner, R. K., Givens, J. E., & Pollack, W. S. (2008). "You're so gay!": Do different forms of bullying matter for adolescent males? *School Psychology Review, 37*(2), 160–173.

Szalacha, L A. (2003). Safer sexual diversity climates: Lessons learned from an evaluation of Massachusetts Safe Schools Program for gay and lesbian students. *American Journal of Education, 110*(1), 58–88.

Szymanski, D. M., Kashubeck-West, S., & Meyer, J. (2008). Internalized heterosexism: A historical and theoretical overview. *The Counseling Psychologist, 36*(4). 510–524.

Talbot, K. (1998–99). Mothers now childless: Personal transformations after the death of an only child. *Omega, 38*(3): 167–186.

Tawake, S. (2006). Cultural rhetoric in coming-out narratives: Witi Ihimaera's The Uncle's Story. *World Englishes, 25*(3/4), 373–380.

Testa, R. J., Sciacca, L. M., Wang, F., Hendricks, M. L., Goldblum, P., Bradford, J., & Bongar, B. (2012). Effects of violence on transgender people. *American Psychological Association, 43*(5), 452–459.

Thane, P. (1998). The family lives of old people. *Old age from antiquity to post-modernity*. New York: Routledge.

The World Professional Association for Transgender Health. (2013). *Standards of care for the health of transsexual, transgender, and gender nonconforming people.* Retrieved from http://www.wpath.org/documents/Standards%20of%20Care%20V7%20-%202011%20WPATH.pdf.

Thompson, C. (2005). *Making parents: The ontological choreography of reproductive technologies.* Cambridge, MA: MIT Press.

Tiemann, K. A., Kennedy, S. A., & Haga, M. P. (1998). Rural lesbians' strategies for coming out to health care professionals. *Journal of Lesbian Studies, 2*(1), 61–75.

Ting-Toomey, S. S. (2005). Identity negotiation theory: Crossing cultural boundaries. In W. B. Gudykunst (Ed.), *Theorizing about intercultural communication* (pp. 211–233). Thousand Oaks, CA: Sage.

Toomey, R. B., Ryan, C., Diaz, R. M., Card, N. A., & Russell, S. T. (2010). Gender-nonconforming lesbian, gay, bisexual, and transgender youth: School victimization and young adult psychosocial adjustment. *Developmental Psychology, 46*(6), 1580–1589.

Troiden, R. R. (1988). Homosexual identity development. *Journal of Adolescent Health Care, 9*(2), 105–113.

Troiden, R. R. (1989). The formation of homosexual identities. *Journal of Homosexuality, 17*(1–2), 43–73.

Tumolo, M. (2011). On useful rhetorical history. *Journal of Contemporary Rhetoric, 1*(2), 55–62.

United States Census Bureau. (2013). *ACS health insurance definitions.* Retrieved from http://www.census.gov/hhes/www/hlthins/methodology/definitions/acs.html.

United States Department of Health and Human Services. (2010). *Healthy people 2020.* Washington, DC: U.S. Department of Health and Human Services. Retrieved from http://healthypeople.gov/2020/topicsobjectives2020/overview.aspx?topicId=25.

United States Department of Health and Human Services. (2010, November 27). *Medicare finalizes new rules to require equal visitation rights for all hospital patients.* HHS.gov. Retrieved from http://www.hhs.gov/news/press/2010pres/11/20101117a.html.

United States Department of Health and Human Services. (2011). *Affordable Care Act to improve data collection, reduce health disparities.* Retrieved from http://www.hhs.gov/news/press/2011pres/06/20110629a.html.

United States Department of Health and Human Services. (2012). HHS LGBT Issues Coordinating Committee 2012 report. *HHS.gov.* Retrieved from http://www.hhs.gov/secretary/about/lgbthealth_objectives_2012.html.

United States General Accounting Office. (1997). *Defense of Marriage Act: Update to prior report* (GAO-04–353R Defense of Marriage Act). Washington, DC. Retrieved from http://www.gao.gov/new.items/d04353r.pdf.

United States v. Windsor, 000 U.S. 12–307 (2013).

Vidal-Ortiz, S. (2009). The figure of the transwoman of color through the lens of 'Doing Gender.' *Gender & Society 23*(10), 99–103.

Vieth, W., & Jaworski, D. (2013, July 20). *Oklahoma Watch study identifies jobs with largest number of uninsured.* Oklahoma Watch. Retrieved from http://oklahomawatch.org/2013/07/20/oklahoma-watch-study-identifies-jobs-with-most-uninsured-workers/.

Vyas, A., Mitra, R., Rao, B. S. S., & Chattarji, S. (2002). Chronic stress induces contrasting patterns of dendritic remodeling in hippocampal and amygdaloid neurons. *The Journal of Neuroscience, 22*(15), 6810–6818.

Wetzstein, C. (2013, August 12). California enacts nation's first law protecting transgender students. *The Washington Times.* Retrieved from http://www.washingtontimes.com/news/2013/aug/12/california-enact-nations-first-law-protecting-tran/.

White, J. C., & Dull, V. T. (1997). Health risk factors and health-seeking behavior in lesbians. *Journal of Women's Health, 6*(1), 103–112.

White, J. C., & Levinson, W. (1995). Lesbian health care: What a primary care physician needs to know. *Western Journal of Medicine, 162,* 463–465.

Wilkerson, A. (1994). Homophobia and the moral authority of medicine. *Journal of Homosexuality, 27*(3–4), 329–347.

Wilkinson, W. (2006). Public health gains of the transgender community in San Francisco: Grassroots organizing and community-based research. In P. Currah, R. M. Juang & S. P. Minter (Eds.), *Transgender rights.* Minneapolis, MN: University of Minnesota Press.

Williams, W. L. (1986). *Spirit and the flesh: Sexual diversity in American Indian culture.* Boston: Beacon Press.

Willingham, T., (2013). The stats on Internet pornography. *Daily Infographic.* Retrieved from http://dailyinfographic.com.

Wingood, G. M., DiClemente, R. J., & Raj, A. (2000). Adverse consequences of intimate partner abuse among women in non-urban domestic violence shelters. *American Journal of Preventive Medicine, 19*(4), 270–275.

Winter, C. (2012). *Responding to LGBT health disparities.* Special Health Equity Series Report by the Missouri Foundation for Health. St Louis, Missouri (pp. 1–39).

Wolkenstein, B. H., & Sterman, L. (1998). Unmet needs of older women in a clinic population: The discovery of possible long-term sequelae of domestic violence. *Professional Psychology: Research and Practice, 29*(4), 341–348.

Wood, J. (2011). *Gendered lives: Gender, communication, and culture.* (9th ed.). Belmont, CA: Wadsworth.

World Health Organization. (2004). *Terminology information system* [online glossary]. Retrieved from http://www.who.int/health-systems-performance/docs/glossary.htm.

Young, E. A., & Akil, H. (1985). Corticotropin-releasing factor stimulation of adrenocorticotropin and beta-endorphin release: Effects of acute and chronic stress. *Endocrinology, 117*(1). 12–30.

Zahnd, E., Grant, D., Aydin, M. J., Chia, J. Y., & Padilla-Frausto, I. D. (2010). *Nearly four million California adults are victims of intimate partner violence.* Policy Brief, UCLA Center for Health Policy Research. Los Angeles, CA. Retrieved from http://healthpolicy.ucla.edu/publications/Documents/PDF/Nearly%20Four%20Million%20California%20Adults%20Are%20Victims%20of%20Intimate%20Partner%20Violence.pdf.

Index

About the Contributors

Mike Allen is professor of communication at the University of Wisconsin-Milwaukee. Dr. Allen received his PhD from Michigan State University. His teaching and research interests include sexuality, persuasion, argumentation, social influence, and research methods. Dr. Allen has been ranked in the top twenty-five of active research career scholars based on the number of published works.

Gina Castle Bell is assistant professor in the Department of Communication Studies at West Chester University. Her research interests are in intercultural communication, with an emphasis on black and white communication, as well as human communication theory, research methods, and research methodology. Dr. Castle Bell received her MA in Interpersonal communication from the University of Central Florida. She earned her PhD in communication studies from George Mason University in 2012.

Bethany Coston is a PhD candidate at Stony Brook University. Her work on masculinities, sexualities, violence, and health have been published in peer-reviewed journals, edited volumes, and special reports; she is also the coeditor of textbooks and readers *Sociology Now, The Gendered Society,* and *Sexualities: Identities, Behavior, and Society.* Her current work is on the dynamic processes of power and inequality on queer intimate partner violence.

Gilbert Gonzales is a PhD candidate in the Division of Health Policy and Management and a research assistant at the State Health Access Data Assistance Center (SHADAC) at the University of Minnesota. Mr. Gonzales's current area of research includes reform efforts to improve health insurance coverage for vulnerable families and children, including same-sex households. His work has appeared in the *American Journal of Public Health and Pediatrics.*

Vickie L. Harvey (PhD, University of Denver) is professor of communication studies at California State University, Stanislaus. Her research in cross-sex friendship and technology has appeared in *Sex Roles, Communication Teacher, International Journal of Information* and *Communication Technology Education,* among others. She and Teresa Heinz Housel have coedited two books on first-generation college students and are currently writing a magazine production textbook.

Teresa Heinz Housel (PhD, Indiana University) is associate professor of communication at Hope College. Her research in homelessness, the politics of housing, media and globalization, alternative media, and language, power, and class have appeared in *Critical Studies in Media Communication, Information, communication & Society,* and *Journal of Critical Inquiry.* She has coedited two books on first-generation college students with Vickie L. Harvey.

Reese Kelley, a white, queer, trans man, holds a PhD in sociology from the University at Albany, SUNY, and is a recipient of the Woodrow Wilson Foundation's Women's and Gender Studies Dissertation Fellowship and the Middlebury College Dissertation and Postdoctoral Fellowships. His research examines the strategies trans people use to achieve inter-, intra-, and/or administrative recognition when confronting cis-normative spaces, policies, and practices.

Miriam King, PhD, is a demographer and historian who has studied living arrangements, fertility differentials, the social construction of population problems, and the history of the U.S. Census. As a research associate at the Minnesota Population Center, she has directed projects to create integrated versions of the Current Population Survey, the U.S. National Health Interview Survey, and the Demographic and Health Surveys.

Gary L. Kreps (PhD, University of Southern California) is a University Distinguished Professor at George Mason University, where he also directs the Center for Health and Risk Communication. He examines the ways strategic interpersonal and mediated communication can enhance health promotion, risk prevention, health advocacy, and quality of care, especially for vulnerable populations. His work is published in more than 380 books, articles, and chapters.

Jimmie Manning (PhD, University of Kansas) is associate professor of communication at Northern Illinois University. His research focuses on relational discourses, especially those about sexuality, gender, love, and identity; connections between relationships and efficacy in health and organizational contexts; and new media. His research has been supported by funding agencies such as the National Science Foundation, and he has accrued more than sixty publications.

Ryan Moltz is a PhD candidate in sociology at the University of Minnesota. He studies human rights, law, and political change and has presented on the effects of evolving HIV testing policies at the International AIDS Conference and the Population Association of America annual meetings. As a research assistant at the Minnesota Population Center, he has worked to integrate data from the National Health Interview Survey.

Sonny Nordmarken is a doctoral candidate in sociology at the University of Massachusetts, Amherst and holds a MA in sexuality studies from San Francisco State University. His dissertation examines emotions and power produced in trans people's everyday interactions, and his piece, "Becoming Ever More Monstrous: Feeling Transgender In-Betweenness" (*Qualitative Inquiry,* December 2013), is forthcoming.

Allan D. Peterkin, MD, is associate professor of psychiatry at the University of Toronto, where he heads the Program in Health, Arts, and Humanities and is the Humanities Lead for Undergraduate Medical Education. His books on cultural history, sexuality, and medicine include *Caring for Lesbian and Gay people-A Clinical Guide* (with Dr. Cathy Risdon). At Mount Sinai Hospital, he has coled therapeutic writing groups for men and women living with HIV and edited a collection of their stories, *STILL HERE—A post-cocktail AIDS anthology.*

Katy Ross (BS, East Carolina University, 2012) is a current master's candidate at Texas Tech University in the Communication Studies Department. She is focusing her studies on transgender culture in the areas of health, interpersonal relations, employment, and identity, among others. She would like to thank Dr. Juliann Scholl and Dr. Gina Castle Bell for the contributions to this study and the continuous support to further her studies.

Juliann C. Scholl (PhD, University of Oklahoma, 2000) is associate professor of communication studies at Texas Tech University. Much of her research emphasizes health care communication and crisis management. Dr. Scholl currently teaches undergraduate and graduate courses in leadership, organizational communication, business and professional communication, small-group communication, health communication, and training and instruction.

Marc J. Silva is a behavioral tutor with four years' experience in applied behavioral analysis, discrete trial training, and one-on-one early intensive behavioral therapy. He has his bachelor of arts in psychology from California State University, Stanislaus. He has done research in human sexuality, and is currently doing research in polyamory and nonmonogamous relationships.

Fredrick Smiley, PhD, is professor of education at Montana State University-Northern, teaching foundations, culture/diversity, and special education. He created "HILTIP," an online teaching methods journal for K–12 educators and their students. He is a contributing reviewer/editor to *Thought and Action*, *The Rural Educator*, *Action in Teacher Education*, and *Journal of Excellence in College Teaching*. He is also writing his third book of poetry.

Dawn L. Strongin is professor of psychology at California State University, Stanislaus. She earned her PhD in applied statistics and research methods with an emphasis in neuropsychology and a minor in educational psychology in 2001. She teaches predominantly neuroscience-related courses. Her primary research areas include preclinical symptoms of Alzheimer's disease, and effects of chronic stressors on cognitive performance and decision making.

Michael Warren Tumolo earned his PhD in communication arts and sciences from Pennsylvania State University. His research interests lie at the intersection between rhetoric, power, and cultural consciousness. His recent scholarship includes work on epideictic rhetoric, political communication, and how empathy may be used as a rhetorical strategy to create a humanizing stance towards LGBT rights.

Alicia VandeVusse is a PhD student in sociology at the University of Chicago. Her research focuses on processes of medicalization, notions of family, and issues of reproduction. Her dissertation explores the formation of "nontraditional" families using assisted reproduction in Germany and the United States, with a focus on how legal and professional regulation (or lack thereof) affects the experiences of patients and providers.

Karina Willes is a doctoral student in communication at the University of Wisconsin-Milwaukee. Ms. Willes obtained her MBA from the University of Wisconsin-Oshkosh in 1999. She is focused on research in the areas of LGBT, technology, and health communication. Her area of specific research interest is doctor-patient communication issues between lesbian patients and doctors.

Lightning Source UK Ltd.
Milton Keynes UK
UKHW022343021121
393270UK00007B/632